Psychotherapy in Later Life

Psychotherapy in Later Life

Edited by

Rajesh R. Tampi
Cleveland Clinic Lerner College of Medicine
of Case Western Reserve University

Brandon C. Yarns
VA Greater Los Angeles Healthcare System

Kristina F. Zdanys
University of Connecticut School of Medicine

Deena J. Tampi
Diamond Healthcare Corporation

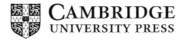
CAMBRIDGE
UNIVERSITY PRESS

CAMBRIDGE
UNIVERSITY PRESS

University Printing House, Cambridge CB2 8BS, United Kingdom

One Liberty Plaza, 20th Floor, New York, NY 10006, USA

477 Williamstown Road, Port Melbourne, VIC 3207, Australia

314–321, 3rd Floor, Plot 3, Splendor Forum, Jasola District Centre, New Delhi – 110025, India

79 Anson Road, #06–04/06, Singapore 079906

Cambridge University Press is part of the University of Cambridge.

It furthers the University's mission by disseminating knowledge in the pursuit of education, learning, and research at the highest international levels of excellence.

www.cambridge.org
Information on this title: www.cambridge.org/9781108701891
DOI: 10.1017/9781108693905

© Cambridge University Press 2020

First published 2020

Printed in the United Kingdom by TJ International Ltd, Padstow Cornwall.

A catalogue record for this publication is available from the British Library.

ISBN 978-1-108-70189-1 Paperback

Contents

Contributors

Deepti Anbarasan

Ali Abbas Asghar-Ali

Meera Balasubramaniam

Patricia Bamonti

Karen M. Benson

Philip Blumenshine

Paul Campion

Patricia Coughlin

Nery Diaz

Christine Dozier

Tyler Durns

Erica Garcia-Pittman

James Gerhart

Victor Gonzalez

M. Lindsey Jacobs

Neha Jain

Pallavi Joshi

Renz J. Juaneza

Cynthia A. Kraus-Schuman

Feyza Marouf

Mark D. Miller

Paroma Mitra

Richard K. Morycz

Brittany A. Mosser

Sarah A. Nguyen

Boski Patel

Patrick J. Raue

Brenna N. Renn

Melissa L. Sanchez

Sandra Swantek

Danielle Tolton

Anh-Thu Tran

Brandon C. Yarns

Foreword

The older I become, the more acutely aware I am of both the overt and covert, dramatic and subtle ways that ageism injures older adults and diminishes their quality of life. Whenever the moment calls for a quick and powerful antidote for the toxicity of ageism, my favorite is an often-cited quote attributed to Henry Wadsworth Longfellow:

> For age is opportunity no less than youth itself, though in another dress, and as the evening twilight fades away, the sky is filled with stars invisible by day.

As a geriatric psychiatrist, psychotherapy practitioner, and professor of psychiatry at the University of California, over the past 30 years I have witnessed first-hand the impact of ageist beliefs and actions on the lives of countless patients in whose care I have participated. One of my greatest disappointments has been appreciating how the adage "You can't teach an old dog new tricks" remains so deeply imbedded in our culture. When teaching students, residents, fellows, and colleagues, I repeat, as often as circumstances permit, that in my opinion there are only three essential ingredients required for successful psychotherapy: some degree of preserved ability to learn, motivation to change, and access to a coach, which could take the form of a self-help book, a trained therapist, or the combination of these two. I emphasize that none of these criteria has anything to do with chronological age. With this in mind, I was both delighted and honored when Raj Tampi and his coeditors, all of whom are highly respected colleagues as well as dear friends, asked me to write this foreword.

Along with the group of talented and accomplished geriatric mental health experts whom they engaged to help them with this project, they have created an invaluable resource for those whose work includes addressing the mental health needs of older adults. As someone who recently turned 60, and by the account of many should have put aside my adolescent idealism, I still hold up the utopian belief that ageism, whether directed toward those who are old or those who are young, has no place in our world. I am deeply gratified to note that the experienced editors and expert authors of this book span the entire spectrum of career stage. Regardless of age or career stage, it deserves mention that some of the authors have acquired firsthand experience with the psychotherapeutic challenges about which they are writing, as both providers of care and recipients of care. This depth of experience is reflected in the accurate perspectives and compassionate tone that inform their writing. In a similar manner, as someone who has spent my entire career working as a member of an interprofessional clinical team, I am also deeply gratified by the diversity in discipline and specialty reflected in those who contributed to this effort. Its varying perspectives form another significant strength of this book.

Although a few other books on this topic have been written over the past 20 years, none is as thoughtfully organized, comprehensive, well researched, and up-to-date as this addition to the literature. The authors clearly outline the indications for psychotherapy as well as provide guidance for choosing among the various psychotherapy modalities. This textbook, unlike others in this area, covers each of the major schools of psychotherapy. In addition, Raj and his coeditors have recognized the importance of including a number of special topics in their book, such as the value of providing psychotherapy to those living with cognitive deficits and the adaptations that facilitate successful outcomes with this subgroup of patients; the role of diversity when providing psychotherapy to older adults, including factors that may be more important than the specific modality of therapy being provided; and the unique psychosocial concerns of and opportunities for patients approaching the end of life. In addition, I especially appreciate the chapter on combining psychotherapy and medication interventions. Given the clinical complexity encountered when working with many older adults, using all of the tools in our toolbox is essential. Even for practitioners who limit their interventions to only pharmacologic or only psychotherapeutic, the knowledge contained in this book will benefit older patients by helping mental health care providers both coordinate and reinforce each other's efforts.

Daniel D. Sewell, MD, DFAPA, DFAAGP
Professor of Clinical Psychiatry
Associate Vice Chair for Geriatric Psychiatry and Development
Codirector of the Division of Geriatric Psychiatry and
Codirector of the Memory Aging and Resilience Clinic
Department of Psychiatry
University of California, San Diego
and
Past President, American Association for Geriatric Psychiatry 2016

Preface

The United Nations reports that between 2017 and 2050, the number of the world's adults older than age 60 is expected to double to approximately 2.1 billion.[1] It is also estimated that over 15% of older adults suffer from a psychiatric disorder.[2] There is a great need for evidence-based treatments specific to later life, as physical and psychological aging, medical comorbidity, unique psychosocial stressors, and other challenges affect the presentation of psychiatric disorders and the suitability of treatment approaches for this population. A significant proportion of the medical literature focuses on pharmacotherapy for psychiatric disorders among older adults. However, there is substantial data highlighting the efficacy of psychotherapy among older adults and the acceptability and tolerability of psychotherapy over pharmacotherapy in this group as well. Drs. Tampi, Yarns, and Zdanys, together with Ms. Tampi, recognized the need to concisely synthesize available evidence and provide a stimulus for wider implementation of psychotherapy for the treatment of older adults, and thus *Psychotherapy in Later Life* was developed.

Organized into chapters by treatment modality and/or target population, the text may be read as a whole to better understand the use of psychotherapy in older adults conceptually or may be approached as a reference by which a specific chapter may begin to inform the implementation of a particular form of psychotherapy in clinical practice. Authors include geriatric psychiatrists and psychologists, among whom some focus their clinical work in psychotherapy, others incorporate psychotherapeutic techniques into a medication-management model, and others conduct research in psychotherapy in later life. The text intends to serve as a resource for anyone who wishes to expand their knowledge base and skill set in the practice of psychotherapy with older adults.

The editors would like to acknowledge their respective mentors, colleagues, trainees, staff, and families for their support and thank all the contributors for their efforts in creating this book.

References

1. United Nations. *World population prospects: the 2017 revision*. New York: United Nations; 2017. ST/ESA/SER.A/399.

2. World Health Organization. *Mental health of older adults*. 2017. Retrieved from: www.who.int/news-room/fact-sheets/detail/mental-health-of-older-adults

Introduction to Psychotherapy with Adults in Later Life

Victor Gonzalez, Erica Garcia-Pittman, Anh-Thu Tran, and Christine Dozier

Introduction

Psychotherapy is an evidence-based treatment for adults in later life with a wide variety of conditions. Simply defined, psychotherapy is the treatment of a mental disorder by psychological rather than medical means. Initial skepticism regarding the use of psychotherapy in older adults rapidly gave way as the quality of psychotherapeutic intervention improved and practitioners better understood and refined themes related to aging.[1] From the 1980s onward, the evidence base for psychotherapy in older adults has continued to grow. Today, theory and evidence show that psychotherapy is indeed an effective treatment for a variety of conditions in older adults. In this chapter, we will review the history of psychotherapy in older adults, provide an overview of the recent evidence supporting its use, outline special issues in conducting psychotherapy with older adults, and introduce the remaining chapters of the book.

History of Psychotherapy for Adults in Later Life

In the early 1900s, Freud's initial theories focused on the influence of childhood on an adult's current life. While his early work focused on patients under the age of fifty,[2] his later writings recognized the treatment potential of psychotherapy for older patients. For example, his paper "Mourning and Melancholia" outlines the treatment of depression in an older population.[3] Jung, a subsequent pioneer in the field of psychoanalysis, further explored work with older adults. He wrote about the stages of life, including childhood, maturity, middle age, and old age.[4] Jung observed that some will reach the final stage with the perspective of having "too much unlived life . . . so that they approach the threshold of old age with unsatisfied demands."[4] He also wrote of the importance in later life of going through an "introspective and self-reflective experience" that involves "searching for and coming to terms with who one is, both individually and collectively."[5]

Later practitioners expanded on early theory by further describing phases of human development. In the 1950s, Erikson outlined such developmental phases of life, with later life being dominated by the issue of ego integrity versus despair.[6] Ego integrity is achieved when people view their life's accomplishments as successful. Alternatively, despair may develop if life is viewed as useless or unaccomplished, or if discontent exists regarding the way past life events took place.

In the 1980s, Colarusso, Nemiroff, and Hildebrand placed greater emphasis on later life in their examination of developmental phases. Colarusso and Nemiroff wrote of developmental tasks in adulthood that included the ongoing evolution and use of psychic structure (rather than its formation alone) and a growing awareness of one's own death. They also emphasized that, in addition to childhood events, past events in young or middle adulthood could influence developmental processes.[7] Themes of "developmental tasks and difficulties in later life" by Hildebrand are dominated by loss, including loss of sexual potency, loss of productivity in work roles, failure of health, loss of potential to achieve going forward, failure as a parent, loss of partner, and one's own death in terms of narcissistic loss and pain.[8]

The work to define phases of human development gave further guidance to therapists working with older adults, as the theory gave a framework for greater understanding of themes related to aging. Despite the initial conception of psychoanalysis as a tool merely for addressing issues related to childhood, researchers and practitioners today recognize that psychotherapeutic intervention is effective for people in all phases of life, including older adults.

The Evolution of Research Supporting Psychotherapy for Adults in Later Life

As psychotherapy theories evolved to acknowledge that therapeutic interventions were beneficial to older adults, researchers began focusing on the effectiveness of therapy in older adults. Advances in research over the last several decades have supported psychotherapeutic approaches as viable treatment options for older adults. However, this has not always been the case. Throughout most of the twentieth century, research on psychotherapy for older adults was lacking because of a bias among researchers that older adults were less likely to seek psychological support than their younger counterparts due to factors including perceived stigma, the assumption that depression and anxiety were part of aging or due to physical ailments, and the perception from older individuals that they could not experience significant changes from psychotherapy.[9,10] Unfortunately, the lack of early empirical research supporting psychotherapy's effectiveness was reflected in national guidelines, such as the 1991 National Institutes of Health (NIH) recommendations on the treatment for depression in older adults. This report listed psychotherapy as a third-line intervention, with pharmacotherapy and electroconvulsive therapy being first and second line treatments, respectively.[11,12] Attitudes toward psychotherapy have since been more positive, thanks in part to more contemporary research studies that have suggested various ways in which psychotherapy can potentially be effective in the treatment of older adults and have provided insight into why psychotherapy is more acceptable as a treatment option by our current aging population.[13]

Over the last several decades, research has consistently shown the positive effects that psychotherapy can have on older adults with mental health needs, including the notion that psychotherapeutic interventions with older adults have a positive effect on the overall improvement of general psychological wellbeing.[13] The benefits that various forms of psychotherapy can produce in older adults with common psychiatric disorders such as depression and anxiety are now well documented.[14] In the case of geriatric depression, meta-analyses have shown that several therapy modalities, including cognitive behavioral therapy (CBT), reminiscence therapy (RT), interpersonal psychotherapy (IPT), and brief dynamic psychotherapy (BDP) are efficacious in treating major depression.[10,15,16] More specifically, research has highlighted several mechanisms by which psychotherapy can be helpful for patients with depression, such as helping to improve coping skills, managing interpersonal stressors, and bolstering social supports.[17,18]

As with depression, psychotherapy has also led to improvement in symptoms in older adults experiencing anxiety. The modalities with the most evidence of effectively treating anxiety for older adults are relaxation training, CBT, and supportive and cognitive therapies.[19,20] Psychotherapy is also a promising treatment option for mental health disorders beyond depression and anxiety. Studies have also shown that psychotherapy can be helpful in older adults diagnosed with schizophrenia, as well as in patients experiencing common geriatric conditions such as insomnia and pain from undergoing medical treatments.[14,21–23]

Not only has research shown psychotherapy's effectiveness for various mental illnesses in older adults, it has contributed to the notion that older adults are more receptive to psychotherapy than was previously believed. Research now suggests that in some instances older adults prefer psychotherapy over pharmacotherapy.[24] Psychotherapy is often preferred over pharmacotherapy because older adults tend to be more sensitive to medications, especially in the context of polypharmacy. Psychotherapeutic interventions can have the added benefit of potentially reducing the medication burden among older adults, which can further help avoid or minimize unfavorable side effects from medications, as well as reduce the risk of falls, cognitive decline, and other medical problems.[20]

More recent research for psychotherapy has focused not only on identifying ways in which it can be a useful treatment tool but also on making it more accessible. Studies have noted that upcoming generations of older adults experience a higher prevalence of depression and other mental disorders than previous generations, driving the need for improved access to psychotherapy.[25] Several exciting efforts utilizing integrated care management systems to facilitate access to mental health care needs in older adults include Primary Care Research in Substance Abuse and Mental Health for the Elderly (PRISM-E);[26] Improving Mood: Promoting Access to Collaborative Treatment (IMPACT);[27] Prevention of Suicide in Primary Care Elderly: Collaborative Trial (PROSPECT);[28] Re-engineering Systems for Primary Care Treatment of Depression (RESPECT-Depression);[29] and the Veterans Administration's (VA's) Unified Psychogeriatric Biopsychosocial Evaluation and Treatment (UPBEAT)[30] program. The goal of these endeavors and future research is to make psychotherapy more accessible in order to further its positive effects in the treatment of older adults.

Considerations for Psychotherapy in Adults in Later Life

Throughout this book, the authors discuss the benefits of psychotherapy and the different modalities to be considered in older adults. Interwoven in these discussions are the special considerations for conducting psychotherapy in this population that require the therapist's awareness. These varied factors will likely become apparent in the process of therapy; however, the most prevalent differences have been outlined by the contextual, cohort-based, maturity, and specific challenge model (CCMSC) laid out by Bob Knight.[31] This model provides a framework for the various considerations and adaptations of therapy in older adults. Refer below to Table 1.1 for an outline of the factors comprising the CCMSC model.

Firstly, in this model, *context* refers to the patient's social and environmental community. Providers should understand that older patients experience a wide range of residential settings, including living independently or in senior living communities, assisted living facilities, nursing homes, locked skilled nursing homes, or even in hospitals. Different environments lead to differences in the challenges that patients face, and thus a detailed knowledge of these settings aid in greater understanding of the patient. For example, a patient in a senior living facility that has little in the way of social activities may struggle more with feelings of isolation and loneliness. Relationships with facility staff or coresidents

Table 1.1 Summary of Bob Knight's Contextual, Cohort-Based, Maturity, and Specific Challenge (CCMSC) Model

Context	Cohort-based (generational) differences	Maturity	Specific challenges (to the aging population)
Living environment -Independent living -Assisted living -Nursing homes -Medical settings	Personality differences Differences in education level	Slowing cognitive processing and declining memory Hearing loss	Chronic illnesses Disabilities Losses and grieving
Social community -Social services -Community-based programs	Differences in values Sociohistorical life experiences	Emotional complexity Experience/expertise	Changing purpose/ identity

can also have a large impact on treatment. Social context also includes community-based programs patients can be involved in, whether it be outside the home (i.e., senior community centers) or inside the home (i.e., inhome health services). Knowledge of the types of resources available in one's community can be beneficial in creating a strong base for referrals to aid with patients' varying needs.[32] Additionally, it is important to be cognizant of the patient's caregivers, family, and friends, as these are the patient's support network outside of therapy. For instance, a patient who has limited relationships may struggle more with depression than someone with a robust support system.

Another significant point when considering an older adult's context is to keep in mind where they tend to seek treatment. Different contexts in which treatment takes place may make the patient more comfortable and open. For example, older adults are more likely to become involved in mental health treatment if it is embedded within primary care rather than offered by mental health clinics,[33] suggesting that integrated health services may improve access to mental health. Thus, having greater knowledge of older adults' preferences for where they receive services can be a way to improve access to psychotherapy for this population.

The second point in the model refers to the cohort differences in this population. While the older adult population was once conceptualized as a homogeneous population with similar issues and psychological mindedness, generational factors (i.e., the Depression-era generation versus the GI generation versus the Baby Boomers) have increasingly been shown to be important. Being more informed about these cohort differences can allow the therapist to better tailor therapy to the patient's needs. For example, in the United States, later-born cohorts have been shown to have had more years of formal schooling than younger-born cohorts.[34] Personality differences have also been seen between generations; in the cohort from the 1900s to World War I, there was decreased extraversion followed by increased extraversion in later cohorts.[32] Changes in social norms across generations play a large role in the experiences of the patient. Understanding these generational differences in social norms involves being more familiar with the historical context that may have shaped the patient's development. For example, a woman who decided to forego having a family for a career in the 1940s could experience a large difference in the psychological impact of that decision compared to a woman who did the same in the 1970s. The therapist may conceptualize the patient differently depending on the patient's generation, education level, and historical context.

The third point in the CCMSC model refers to maturation, which relates to the process of aging itself. The process of psychotherapy may be affected by developmental maturation to varying degrees. Firstly, maturation can lead to greater wisdom or a greater depth of knowledge in the patient, which may make therapy more robust. That older adults will have had more experience may be a great strength. Therefore, rather than exploring new skills as one would for a young patient, tapping into the strengths that already exist in the older patient may be an important approach. Similarly, greater depth to emotional complexity may occur with aging.[31] Older patients may understand and solve problems in different ways than therapists would expect, as they may not have had the robust experiences that their patients have had. A younger therapist may find it difficult to fully understand the views of the older patient. However, if we allow ourselves to learn from the patient, these nuances may be enlightening and may even aid in our development as therapists. Thus, maturation can change therapy in a variety of ways that require flexibility from and even growth in the therapist.

Other changes that may occur in some older adults are diminished cognitive processing speed and memory. Slower cognitive processing may require the therapist to slow down the pace of the session or use simpler language. Short-term memory may decline due to normal aging or a neurocognitive disorder. Although psychotherapy is possible with these patients, the therapist will have to be more patient and flexible when patients are discussing their worries and concerns. Using notes and reminders may also be useful when interacting with patients with cognitive decline, and being more cognizant of such minor adjustments as speaking more clearly and slowly may help patients with hearing loss.[32]

The final point in the model considers the challenges and issues older adults struggle with that are specific to that portion of life. As patients age, chronic illnesses, disability, and losses become more and more prevalent and are often prominent topics in therapy. Medical illnesses may precipitate psychological struggles, and psychological issues may exacerbate physical symptoms/illnesses or even be masked as medical symptoms. Parceling out psychological symptoms and physical symptoms can be difficult for providers, and thus knowledge about patients' illnesses can become vital. For example, intermittent palpitations could be a signal of anxiety in a patient in good cardiovascular health or a symptom of arrhythmias in a patient with heart failure. Understanding a patient's medical illnesses may help in decision-making while also allowing a better understanding of the challenges the patient faces because of them. With greater knowledge of the patient's specific struggles, the therapist can provide the support a patient needs in these situations.

In addition to illnesses, losses in both the literal sense of losing loved ones and the psychological sense of losing one's abilities or purpose are specific issues that older patients face and for which they need support. Patients seeking treatment for depression frequently have experienced several losses in the preceding months or years.[31] These losses put patients at risk for complicated grief, which recent evidence shows is underdiagnosed and under-treated, and should be distinguished from major depression.[35] Providers must therefore be prepared to discuss the topics of death and dying to support patients through these difficult times.

Patients may similarly struggle with losses in their lives that may be less tangible, such as a loss of identity or loss of purpose that may occur with retirement and worsening medical conditions. One of the major factors that leads to depression is a loss of independence when transitioning from independent living to an assisted living or nursing home environment.[36] With increasing medical illnesses, patients may also experience additional losses in independence when they must rely more on others for daily functioning. These kinds of losses can be a predominant topic in therapy with some patients.

Though the CCMSC model provides a framework for the important considerations in treating older adults, it also emphasizes the diversity seen in this population. Therapists must learn to adapt their skills and even learn new skills as they embark on the journey to treat older adults. Though some challenges will be met, constant opportunities for growth and learning will also be present.

Psychotherapy for Late-Life Psychiatric Disorders: An Overview

Having established the historical context of psychotherapy and how it relates to older adults, as well as the factors that led to a change in perception toward this intervention, this section of Chapter 1 is an overview of the topics and ideas we convey throughout this book. Overall, our goal is to provide a contemporary summary of various psychotherapy modalities, including the evidence behind them, as well as approaches on how to implement them in the appropriate geriatric patient populations. To this end, the book is divided into three parts:

- Part I provides readers with an overview of psychotherapy, indications for psychotherapy in older adults, and advice on selecting the best modality for an individual patient.
- Part II is a how-to guide for evidence-based psychotherapy approaches. This section focuses on the following four psychotherapy modalities: CBT, problem-solving therapy (PST), IPT, and short-term psychodynamic therapy. The chapters in this section include an introduction of the modality with an overview of the research in support of these therapeutic approaches. They also provide a theoretical framework of each therapy modality along with suggestions on appropriate patient populations. Patient vignettes are utilized in this section to help the reader understand how each psychotherapy approach is applied in practice.
- Part III includes special topics that may arise in psychotherapy. Topics include psychotherapy and cognitive disorders, combined psychotherapy and medication management, psychotherapy with diverse older adults, individual versus group psychotherapy, and psychotherapy at the end of life.

This book aims to educate mental health professionals on the power and significance of psychotherapy and provide tools to help them begin implementing evidence-based psychotherapy into their practices in order to have a positive impact on their patients' lives.

References

1. Garner J. Psychotherapies and older adults. *Aust N Z J Psychiatry*. 2003;37:537.

2. Freud S. Selected papers on hysteria and other psychoneuroses. 1912. Retrieved from: www.bartleby.com/280/8.html (November 30, 2018).

3. Freud S. *General psychological theory: papers on metapsychology*. New York: Touchstone; 1997.

4. Jung CG. Structure and dynamics of the psyche. Adler G, Hull RFC, editors. Princeton, NJ: Princeton University Press; 1970. (*Collected Works of C.G. Jung*; vol 8).

5. Evans S, Garner J. *Talking over the years: a handbook of dynamic psychotherapy with older adults*. New York: Brunner-Routledge; 2004.

6. Erikson E. *Identity and the life cycle*. Revised ed. New York: W. W. Norton; 1994.

7. Colarusso GA, Nemiroff RA. *Adult development: a new dimension in psychodynamic theory and practice*. New York: Plenum; 1981.

8. Hildebrand HP. Psychotherapy with older patients. *Br J Med Psychol*. 1982;55:19–28.

9. Yang JA, Jackson CL. Overcoming obstacles in providing mental health treatment to older adults: getting in the door. *Psychotherapy*. 1998;35(4):498–505.

10. Rybarczyk B, Gallagher-Thompson D, Rodman J, et al. Applying cognitive-behavioral psychotherapy to the chronically ill elderly: treatment issues and case illustration. *Int Psychogeriatr*. 1992;4(1):127–140.

11. NIH Consensus Development Conference. Diagnosis and treatment of depression in late life: November 4–6, 1991. *NIH Consens State Sci Statements*. 1991;9(3):1–27.

12. Mackin RS, Areán PA. Evidence-based psychotherapeutic interventions for geriatric depression. *Psychiatr Clin North Am*. 2005;28(4):805–820.

13. Pinquart M, Sörensen S. How effective are psychotherapeutic and other psychosocial interventions with older adults? A meta-analysis. *J Ment Health Aging*. 2001;7(2):207–243.

14. Gatz M. Commentary on evidence-based psychological treatments for older adults. *Psychol Aging*. 2007;22(1):52–55.

15. Wilson K, Mottram PG, Vassilas C. Psychotherapeutic treatments for older depressed people. *Cochrane Database Syst Rev*. 2008;1:CD004853.

16. Huang AX, Delucchi K, Dunn LB, et al. A systematic review and meta-analysis of psychotherapy for late-life depression. *Am J Geriatr Psychiatry*. 2015;23(3):261–273.

17. Pinquart M, Duberstein PR, Lyness JM. Treatments for later-life depressive conditions: a meta-analytic comparison of pharmacotherapy and psychotherapy. *Am J Psychiatry*. 2006;163(9):1493–1501.

18. Wei W, Sambamoorthi U, Olfson M, et al. Use of psychotherapy for depression in older adults. *Am J Psychiatry*. 2005;162(4):711–717.

19. Wetherell JL, Lenze EJ, Stanley MA. Evidence-based treatment of geriatric anxiety disorders. *Psychiatr Clin North Am*. 2005;28(4):871–896.

20. Ayers CR, Sorrell JT, Thorp SR, et al. Evidence-based psychological treatments for late-life anxiety. *Psychol Aging*. 2007;22(1):8–17.

21. Van Citters AD, Pratt SI, Bartels SJ, et al. Evidence-based review of pharmacologic and nonpharmacologic treatments of older adults with schizophrenia. *Psychiatr Clin N Am*. 2005;28(4):913–939.

22. Berry K, Barrowclough C. The needs of older adults with schizophrenia: implications for psychological interventions. *Clin Psychol Rev*. 2009;29(1):68–76.

23. McCurry SM, Logsdon RG, Teri L, et al. Evidence-based psychological treatments for insomnia in older adults. *Psychol Aging*. 2007;22(1):18–27.

24. Gum AM, Areán PA, Hunkeler E, et al. Depression treatment preferences in older primary care patients. *Gerontologist*. 2006;46(1):14–22.

25. Knight B. Psychotherapy and older adults: resource guide. 2009. Retrieved from: www.apa.org/pi/aging/resources/guides/psychotherapy.aspx (November 10, 2018).

26. Levkoff SE, Chen H, Coakley E, et al. Design and sample characteristics of the PRISM-E multisite randomized trial to improve behavioral health care for the elderly. *J Aging Health*. 2004;16(1):3–27.

27. Unützer J, Katon W, Callahan CM, et al. Collaborative care management of late-life depression in the primary care setting: a randomized controlled trial. *JAMA*. 2002;288(22):2836–2845.

28. Alexopoulos GS, Reynolds CF, Bruce ML, et al. Reducing suicidal ideation and

depression in older primary care patients: 24-month outcomes of the PROSPECT study. *Am J Psychiatry.* 2009;**166**(8): 882–890.

29. Dietrich AJ, Oxman TE, Williams JW, et al. Re-engineering systems for the treatment of depression in primary care: cluster randomized controlled trial. *Br Med J.* 2004;**329**:602–605.

30. Kominski G, Andersen R, Bastani R, et al. UPBEAT: the impact of a psychogeriatric intervention in VA medical centers. *Med Care.* 2001;**39**(5):500–512.

31. Knight BG. Unique aspects of psychotherapy with older adults. In: Qualls S, Knight B, editors. *Psychotherapy for depression in older adults.* Hoboken, NJ: John Wiley & Sons; 2006. p. 3–28.

32. Zarit SH, Knight BG. Psychotherapy and aging: multiple strategies, positive outcomes. In: Zarit S, Knight B, editors. *A guide to psychotherapy and aging: effective clinical interventions in a late-stage context.* Washington, DC: American Psychological Association; 1996. p. 1–13.

33. Bartels SJ, Coakley EH, Zubritsky C, et al. Improving access to geriatric mental health services: a randomized trial comparing treatment engagement with integrated versus enhanced referral care for depression, anxiety, and at-risk alcohol use. *Am J Psychiatry.* 2004;**161**(8): 1455–1462.

34. Schaie KW. Intellectual development in adulthood. In: Birren J, Schaie K, editors. *Handbook of the psychology of aging.* 4th ed. San Diego, CA; 1996. p. 266–286.

35. Supiano KP, Luptak M. Complicated grief in older adults: a randomized controlled trial of complicated grief group therapy. *Gerontologist.* 2013;**54**(5):840–856.

36. Choi NG, Ransom S, Wyllie RJ. Depression in older nursing home residents: the influence of nursing home environmental stressors, coping, and acceptance of group and individual therapy. *Aging Ment Health.* 2008;**12**(5):536–547.

Indications for Psychotherapy in Adults in Later Life

Tyler Durns, Danielle Tolton, Sarah A. Nguyen, and Neha Jain

Introduction

Since its inception more than 100 years ago, theories and techniques of psychotherapy have experienced tremendous growth and diversification. There has been a gradual increase in our knowledge of aging as well as in our experience conducting psychotherapy with older adults. Although the core principles of psychotherapy are mostly similar to those pertaining to younger people, certain challenges and themes are unique to this population. These include a diverse range of living environments as well as an increasing need for social integration, adjusting to functional and cognitive decline, accessing services, caregiving, navigating transitions, and managing acute and chronic conditions.[1] An increasing number of older adults are seeking treatment for a broad array of mental health problems, including depression, anxiety, insomnia, personality disorders, cognitive impairment, chronic pain, and substance use. Depending on the patient and the presenting problem, psychotherapy can be used as either a primary or an adjunctive method of treatment.

The choice of psychotherapeutic treatment depends on a variety of factors: current research and evidence, the therapist's theoretical orientation, and what may work best in the presenting situation. It is important to recognize the factors necessitating psychotherapy for the patient, the goals of treatment, and the patient's ability to participate in a particular therapy modality. Although the current population of older adults experiences higher levels of health and wellbeing than in previous generations, the multitude of later life changes continues to challenge the functioning and resilience of older adults.[2,3]

This chapter will explore the indications for psychotherapy as they relate to specific disorders encountered in later life and the evidence for the modalities suggested. We will also discuss the role of psychotherapy in wellbeing and successful aging for older adults.

Specific Indications for Psychotherapy

Depression

Geriatric depression is a common and debilitating disease. Fortunately, an abundance of evidence supports the efficacy of both pharmacologic and psychotherapeutic modalities for its treatment. Effective psychotherapy modalities include but are not limited to group therapy, psychodynamic therapy, interpersonal psychotherapy (IPT), various forms of cognitive behavioral therapy (CBT), reminiscence therapy (RT), and art and music therapy. Multiple studies over the years have shown that psychotherapies are as effective as medications, and combined treatment can both improve response and enhance its breadth and stability.[4,5] In addition to demonstrating efficacy, psychotherapy has been shown to lead to improvements in brain functioning that correlate with response. For instance, one study by Alexopoulos[6] postulated that behavioral modification could target the dysfunction in brain circuitry that contributes to late-life depression. This study found statistically significant decreases in depressive symptoms as measured by the Hamilton Rating Scale for Depression (HAM-D) with use of positive reinforcements and rewards.[6]

Both individual and group psychotherapy have proved effective for geriatric depression. However, group therapy may provide advantages over individual interventions in regard to both feasibility of and access to treatment in some depressed, advanced-age patients. This has been substantiated in a systematic review of nine studies that demonstrate the advantages of group psychotherapy as an adjunct to individual therapy and/or pharmacologic interventions.[7] There was a significant improvement in HAM-D and Geriatric Depression Scale (GDS) total scores in the group receiving CBT in addition to antidepressant medication compared to those using antidepressants alone after two weeks. Furthermore, compliance with pharmacologic treatment improves with adjunctive group cognitive behavioral therapy.[8] One limitation of group therapy is that it entails multiple confounders, such as the dynamic of the group as well as the approach of the provider.

Cognitive behavioral therapy has proven to be a valuable tool in treating depression at all ages and can be used either as a stand-alone or adjunctive therapy. The efficacy of an antidepressant alone versus CBT alone versus a combination of the two for older adults meeting criteria for major depressive disorder (MDD) has been studied.[9-12] According to most analyses, the combined groups show greater improvement than antidepressant-alone groups, whereas the CBT-alone groups often showed improvement but only marginally so over medication-alone interventions. Combined therapies were most effective in patients who were more severely depressed, particularly when antidepressant medication was at or above recommended stable dosage levels.[5]

Because of continual growth in the population of older adults, the public health burden of late-life depression is increasing, placing increasing demands on geriatric mental health providers. In response, other means of delivering treatment have been investigated. Internet-delivered cognitive behavioral therapy (iCBT) has been shown to be both efficacious and feasible despite predicted technical barriers. Moreover, iCBT was found to be an effective treatment option for depression in later life at similar rates to those in younger adults.[13] Telemedicine has also been investigated as a means to increase access of care for older adults facing barriers of mobility, stigma, and geographical isolation. In a large study, treatment response was found to be non-inferior to in-room psychotherapy in older adults. Subjective measurements and remission according to Structured Clinical Interview for the DSM-IV showed similar response.[14]

Several studies have investigated the utility of RT for depression treatment in older adults.[15,16] Results have varied significantly, with about half of the studies showing that RT resulted in statistically significant decreases in depression.[17] A study by Watt and Cappeliez[18] found that 58% of older adults with depression treated with RT showed improvement in depressive symptoms in a follow-up survey after three months. According to the authors, different techniques are likely responsible for the variability in efficacy, but it should be considered a potentially beneficial treatment.[17]

In addition, IPT has demonstrated effectiveness in treating depression. A study by Bruce and colleagues found lower rates of depression and suicidal ideation (SI) in patients treated with interpersonal psychotherapy.[19] Brief dynamic psychotherapy (BDP) has been shown to be an effective intervention for late-life depression.[20] Supportive psychotherapy may also be beneficial, but several studies have demonstrated the superiority of other psychotherapies, such as problem-solving therapy (PST), when older adults have both depression and executive dysfunction.[21]

Less conventional and newer modalities of psychotherapy for the elderly have been pursued as well. Music therapy three times a week has been shown to decrease depression levels at eight weeks.[22] Geriatric Depression scores also improved with garden therapy (both alone and guided) and art therapy.[23]

Subsyndromal Depression

Characterized as depressive symptoms that do not meet the threshold for MDD, subsyndromal depression (SSD), also called subthreshold depression or mild depression, is an under-diagnosed and growing problem, especially in older adults.[24] With an estimated prevalence rate of 15% in older adults, SSD plays a significant role in many American lives and has significant rates of comorbid affective, anxiety, and personality disorders.[24,25] A data review of more than 10,000 adults over age 55 found that an additional 13.8% met the criteria for SSD beyond the 13.7% of US older adults who met the criteria for major depressive disorder.[24] Subsyndromal depression has been associated with lower quality of life, increased disability, and increased suicide risk.[26]

One of the concerns for SSD is that, if left untreated, up to 20–25% of cases may develop into MDD within a year.[26] Fortunately, several studies have demonstrated the effectiveness of psychotherapy for the treatment of subsyndromal depression. Psychotherapeutic treatments for SSD include cognitive, behavioral, and problem-solving therapy.[27] Reynolds and colleagues found that problem-solving therapy was effective in protecting older adults from developing MDD episodes over a two-year period with an average four-point drop in the Beck Depression Inventory (BDI).[26] Other studies have demonstrated the effectiveness of other therapies, including art therapy, mindfulness-based therapy, and reminiscence therapy.[28]

Anxiety

Although anxiety disorders are among the most prevalent psychiatric disorders in the elderly, they tend to be under-diagnosed and inadequately treated.[29] Care must be taken in regard to pharmaceutical management, as sedative and hypnotic medications carry increased risk of respiratory depression, falls, and other serious potential side effects.[30] Psychotherapeutic interventions should thus be pursued aggressively when supported by evidence.

Multiple meta-analyses have shown that CBT was more successful than matched controls receiving no treatment or treatment as usual (TAU).[31,32] This has been found to be especially true in older persons with panic disorder. Cognitive behavioral therapy was also found to be successful in reducing avoidance behaviors characteristic of many anxiety disorders.[33] There is less robust evidence for CBT in treating generalized anxiety disorder (GAD).[34]

Relaxation training has also been found to successfully reduce symptoms of GAD,[35] and presents an efficacious and low-cost intervention. One review concluded that CBT (alone or augmented with RT) does not have any benefit beyond RT alone.[36] More studies directly comparing RT to CBT, or simply testing RT alone, are needed in the future.

Acceptance and commitment therapy (ACT) has been considered as well in the treatment of generalized anxiety disorder. In a small feasibility study, seven older adults who received ACT showed improvement in anxiety and worry. The effect size was smaller than in younger adults who were shown to respond to ACT more robustly.[37] Mindfulness-based stress reduction (MBSR) is a similar approach in that ACT and MBSR both make use of behavioral skills and emphasize psychological flexibility. These treatments may help older adults cope with life experiences that are nonmodifiable, such as worsening health, loss of loved ones, and changes in identity.[38]

Insomnia

Insomnia is a common health problem with significant psychiatric and medical consequences in older adults. Pharmacotherapy is frequently used in psychiatric settings. However, for older adults, concerns about polypharmacy, challenges pertaining to changing pharmacodynamics, and increased vulnerability to side effects make pharmacotherapy risky. As such, psychotherapeutic interventions should always be considered.

Cognitive behavioral therapy has been shown to be beneficial for older adults with insomnia. Studies have examined the role of CBT for insomnia (CBT-I) in older patients with both primary psychiatric disorders and secondary insomnia from osteoarthritis, coronary artery disease, and pulmonary disease.[39] Cognitive behavioral therapy was found to be more effective when compared to general wellness and basic sleep hygiene interventions.[39] Sleep latency, early morning awakening, and sleep efficiency have all been shown to improve significantly with CBT, both with and without concurrent pharmacologic treatment. Maintenance of symptomatic control has also been demonstrated in long-term follow-up studies utilizing cognitive behavioral therapy.[40]

Brief behavioral treatment for insomnia (BBTI) was also found to be efficacious for chronic insomnia in older adults.[41] This has implications for its use in primary care and medical settings due to its ease of use as a short-term treatment relative to cognitive behavioral therapy.

Personality Disorders

The establishment of approaches to treat personality disorders (PDs) in older adults is a widely acknowledged deficit in all treatment settings. Personality disorders are viewed as compounding factors in the psychopathology of frequently comorbid mood, anxiety, and substance use disorders. Characteristic late-life changes can make older adults particularly vulnerable to the heightened interpersonal disturbance and emotional distress characteristic of many personality disorders. Data generally support the notion that cluster B personality disorders show improvement over time, while the other clusters (A and C) are characterized by a more chronic course and may worsen with age.[42]

As with younger and middle-aged persons, dialectical behavioral therapy (DBT) has been shown to have a positive outcome in treating PDs in the elderly. This is not only true for these disorders alone but also with comorbid depression. Two studies utilizing standard DBT to treat depression and PDs in older adults showed superior results in treating geriatric patients with both diagnoses; HAM-D scores improved compared to medication alone, as well as treatment success in patients who previously failed medications alone.[43] These findings are consistent with those for younger adults, lending further credence to the notion that PDs in the elderly should be approached in a similar manner, even if population-specific studies are lacking.

Schemas, which are enduring ways of viewing the world, are nevertheless dynamic constructs that abate and intensify in accordance with both internal and external factors.

Schema therapy (ST) is an effective therapy for PDs in adults; however, empirical research into ST in older adults specifically is limited. Several small studies have examined this and found ST to be an effective treatment for cluster C PDs in older adults in regard to symptomatic distress and quality-of-life metrics, as well as for improving target complaints.[44]

Cognitive Impairment

The increasing prevalence of cognitive impairment (CI) inherent in normal aging demands that further attention be paid to both pharmacologic and psychotherapeutic treatments. Patients with all forms of CI ranging from mild CI to severe CI must face a multitude of task- and memory-related problems associated with psychosocial dysfunction.

Various modalities in the realm of CBT-based strategies (computerized cognitive training, traditional CBT, cognitive rehabilitation, etc.) have been examined, and all demonstrated significant improvement in cognition and other neuropsychiatric symptoms as demonstrated through the Illness Cognition Questionnaire (ICQ) and various subscales.[45,46] Cognitive behavioral therapy has been found to be effective in significantly altering dysfunctional beliefs and thinking errors associated with CI in as few as 16–20 sessions. On review, CBT was also effective in improving coping skills, actual and perceived agency, and stress management.[47]

Alzheimer's Disease

As the healthcare industry continues to improve in treating fatal illnesses earlier in life, the incidence of Alzheimer's disease (AD) continues to increase, necessitating the understanding and use of psychotherapeutic techniques in its management. This necessity is underscored by the relative dearth of pharmacological and other medical treatments for Alzheimer's disease.

Behavioral and environmental interventions should be used in managing Alzheimer's disease. However, not only are these interventions difficult to standardize but they also show only nonspecific and modest effects.[48] Evidence indicates that families should be heavily involved when possible, with studies involving family caregivers demonstrating improvements in both patient and caregiver quality of life.[49]

Reminiscence therapy is one psychotherapeutic technique used for AD in which participants are encouraged to talk about past events and often journal them. Reminiscence therapy in AD may lead to improvement in cognition and behavioral functioning. Caregiver strain was also found to decrease in those who participated with their afflicted relative.[50] Its effects on mood, cognition, and wellbeing in dementia, however, are less well understood.

Psychotic Disorders

Psychosis often differs both in presentation and etiology in the elderly as compared to other age groups. Evidence supporting the role of psychotherapy in these individuals is limited. While there have been several articles published on psychotherapy for psychotic patients, they predate the advent of many or even all antipsychotic medications. Despite some schools of thought, psychotherapy-centered treatment without primary medication-centered treatment should be viewed as below the standard of care for psychotic disorders. Among primary approaches, CBT is likely the most hopeful in that it has been shown to be of some benefit in young persons with primary psychotic disorders who are stable on medications.[51]

Adjustment Disorders

Another under-diagnosed condition in the older adult population is adjustment disorder. With a higher level of distress than what would be expected for a stressor, adjustment disorder can be significantly detrimental to occupational, social, and educational functioning. As age increases, so does the risk of comorbid medical conditions, disability, and loss of mobility and independence. As the aging population copes with a variety of life changes, many older adults face developing adjustment disorders. Risk factors for adjustment disorder in cancer patients include being female, having lower educational attainment, and metastasis.[52] A meta-analysis found an approximate 6.9% prevalence rate of adjustment disorder after stroke.[53]

A variety of psychotherapies can be employed to treat this condition, including CBT, group-based therapies, and mindfulness; however, psychodynamic psychotherapy in inpatient settings has not been found to be effective given the length of time required.[54] Group psychotherapy was found to decrease SI in adults with adjustment disorders, and mindfulness group therapy was shown to be equally effective as individualized CBT in adult patients.[55,56] Brief supportive psychotherapy has also been demonstrated to be effective in both inpatient and outpatient settings.[57]

Chronic/Complicated Grief

Complicated grief is a debilitating disorder that affects millions of American adults, many of whom are older adults.[58] It occurs in 2–3% of the general population and includes symptoms of longing or emotional pain, inability to accept loss, preoccupying thoughts of the deceased, and intense yearning.[59] Chronic grief is more likely to occur after the loss of a child or life partner, and is highest in women age 60 years and older.[59] Symptoms may persist without treatment, and early intervention and appropriate treatment is key to preventing decreased functioning.[59]

Derived from CBT, motivational interviewing (MI), and IPT, complicated grief treatment (CGT) has been shown to be nearly twice as effective in treatment of complicated grief. In a study by Shear and colleagues, CGT was found to be more effective than interpersonal psychotherapy in adults aged 18–80 for both time to response and response rate of complicated grief.[60] Both CGT and IPT demonstrated effectiveness in treating complicated grief; however, the response rate of CGT was almost twice that of interpersonal psychotherapy.[58]

Few studies have compared psychotherapy with antidepressant treatment for chronic grief. In one such study, the addition of citalopram did not significantly improve the outcome of Clinical Global Impression (CGI) scale measurements when compared with participants who received CGT alone; however, citalopram did appear to optimize treatment of cooccurring depressive symptoms.[61] The addition of psychotropic medication is indicated if comorbid psychiatric diagnoses are present but may not be indicated in the treatment of complicated grief alone.

Chronic Pain

Along with a variety of comorbid medical conditions, chronic pain can be a debilitating problem for many older adults. Chronic pain is prevalent in about 47–63% of adults over the age of 65, and adults over age 50 are twice as likely to be diagnosed with chronic pain.[62,63] Chronic pain can lead to decreased mobility and an increased fear of falling.[64] This in turn can cause an increased risk of depression, physical disability, and limitations in activity and social roles.[64] With a national movement to minimize the prescription of opiates and prevent polypharmacy, psychotherapy techniques are increasingly important in the treatment of chronic pain for improved functioning and quality of life in older adults.[64]

Cognitive behavioral therapy has been the most widely studied psychotherapy and has demonstrated efficacy in the treatment of chronic pain. In one study by Nicholas,[65] patients in the CBT group had better posttreatment outcomes regarding decreased mobility, depressive symptoms, pain-related distress, fear-avoidance beliefs, and self-efficacy for managing pain at one-month follow-up. However, other meta-analyses have shown only modest and short-term benefits.[62]

Preoperative mindfulness-based stress reduction therapy has been linked to improvement in mood and activity in chronic pain patients.[66] Yi found pain scales were decreased in surgical patients who completed mindfulness-based stress reduction.[66] Another study demonstrated improvement in short-term decreases in pain scales after an eight-week mindfulness-based stress reduction.[67] Lastly, multiple studies have demonstrated the effectiveness of biofeedback and relaxation techniques in reducing headaches in older adults, especially when the therapy, including CBT, group-based therapies, and mindfulness, was "tailored to the information processing capacities of the elderly."[68]

Substance Use Disorders

The aging baby boomer cohort has highlighted the often-overlooked presence of alcohol and substance use disorders in older adults, requiring a shift in focus to address the needs of this particular population.[69] Per the 2017 National Survey of Drug Use and Health, 2.8% of adults over the age of 65 reported heavy alcohol use in the past month while 11.5% reported binge alcohol use. Nearly 6% of adults older than 65 years reported using an illicit drug in the past year.[70]

Misuse of prescription and over-the-counter drugs is also becoming more prevalent in this population. The latest data from the National Surveys on Drug Use and Health reveal that 2.2% of adults 65 and older reported misuse of prescription psychotherapeutic drugs while 1.6% reported misuse of opioids.[70]

Over the last two decades, an increasing number of studies has evaluated modified therapies specifically tailored to older adults with substance use disorders. Brief intervention therapies have frequently been studied in the primary care setting. Several clinical trials have shown that 10–30% of problem drinkers have been able to reduce their drinking after brief 1–3-session interventions.[71,72] In one controlled clinical trial, intervention group patients received two 10–15-minute physician-delivered counseling sessions that included advice, education, and contracting using a scripted workbook. The older adults who received the physician intervention demonstrated a significant reduction in seven-day alcohol use, episodes of binge drinking, and frequency of excessive drinking.

Either as a stand-alone therapy or combined with other approaches, CBT seems to be effective in treating alcohol use disorder, both in individual and group settings. In a Veterans Affairs (VA) medical system study, researchers explored outcomes for 12 mixed-age alcohol treatment programs. The programs were oriented partly to CBT, and partly to 12-step and eclectic approaches. Older patients with alcohol use disorders who had gone through the programs were compared with matched groups of younger patients. Older patients had better outcomes than young and middle-aged patients and comparable levels of continuing substance abuse care and 12-step self-help group involvement.[73]

In a residential treatment study, a combination of CBT, MI, and a 12-step approach was used for 67 alcohol-dependent older adults. This study included adaptations for older adults, such as handicapped access, slower program pace, and modifications for vision, hearing, and mild cognitive problems. Special groups included topics such as grief, loss, continuing care, leisure, recreation, and life-stage transitions. Seventy-one percent and 60% of participants were continuously abstinent at 6 and 12 months, respectively.[74]

Motivational interviewing has also been shown to be effective for older adults. In a randomized, double-blind, placebo-controlled efficacy trial of naltrexone for the treatment of alcohol dependence, all subjects received MI-based supportive intervention. Compared with younger adults, older adults had greater attendance at therapy sessions and greater adherence to the medication, resulting in less relapse.[75] Given the adaptability of MI techniques to brief interventions, MI is an ideal intervention for alcohol use disorders in older adults seen in the primary care setting.[76]

Group psychotherapy based upon CBT and MI techniques has also been shown to be effective in the elderly. In a study exploring the outcomes of group therapy in 199 adults older than 50 years, those who completed the program were more likely to reduce nonmedical prescription drug use and to report a reduction in trouble understanding or concentrating due to drug or alcohol use. Completers were also more likely to report improved cognitive functioning, mental health, and vitality, and less bodily pain.[73]

To summarize, multiple psychotherapeutic modalities have been successfully adapted for use in substance use disorders in older adults. In fact, group therapies may be of particular benefit to older adults because of their emphasis on social support.[77] Ideally, all psychotherapeutic interventions, including age-specific adaptations, should be tailored to the patient.

Wellbeing and Successful Aging

Traditionally, aging has been viewed as a period of progressive decline in physical, cognitive, and psychosocial functioning that can lead to a growing healthcare burden on society. Several studies in different countries have examined the role of objective dimensions to predict successful aging, including physical health, social support from family and friends, free-time investment, and physical activity.[1,2] Unfortunately, research advances in understanding successful aging have been challenging given inconsistencies in the literature. For example, 28 studies published on this subject included 29 different definitions of successful aging, with many studies focused primarily on physical health.[2,3] Despite these limitations, psychotherapy can play a key role in enhancing and maintaining the general health and psychological wellbeing of older adults, which can be characterized by three aspects: evaluative wellbeing (or life satisfaction), hedonic wellbeing (feelings of happiness, pleasure, etc.), and eudemonic wellbeing (having a sense of purpose and meaning in life).[78]

To enhance psychological wellbeing, positive psychology has emerged to provide an evidence-based understanding of human flourishing by cultivating positive feelings, positive behaviors, or positive cognitions.[79] Ongoing scientific research, especially in the last decade, suggests that positive traits and the development of interventions that bolster them have the potential to reduce the current and future burden of mental and physical health problems in older adults.[79,80] Studies examining the effectiveness of life review therapy, positive RT, and bibliotherapy have all demonstrated significant improvement in self-esteem, resilience and integrity, life satisfaction, and psychological wellbeing in older adults.[15,81,82]

Problem-solving therapy is effective for modifying behaviors that create poor health outcomes.[83,84] Recent studies have determined that PST is effective in reducing anxiety and depression and increases problem-solving abilities in both community-based and in-home settings.[83] Additionally, consistent support was found for the efficacy of telephone and videophone PST, suggesting these as alternate means of accessing mental health services by homebound elders.[85] In addition to PST, MI has also been found to be effective in older adults with specific health conditions such as heart failure and diabetes.[86,87] Although MI was originally developed to treat substance use disorders, a meta-analysis by Burke et al. demonstrated that MI is equally, if not more, effective as compared to other therapeutic interventions in improving mood and encouraging healthier behaviors including weight loss, increased physical exercise, decreased substance use, and improved pain.[88] A separate study by Heisel also found improved psychological wellbeing as well as decreased suicide rates in older adults over a 16-session course of interpersonal psychotherapy.[89]

To date, there are no reviews of intervention effectiveness for the healthy elderly despite growing interest in the concept of successful aging.[90]

Conclusions

The geriatric population is both vulnerable and often neglected in regard to physical and mental health. Resources are often scarce, and the compounding emotional, physical, and public health costs of these ailments can make appropriate and timely treatment challenging but imperative. With concerns about polypharmacy in increasingly medically complex older adults, the need for nonpharmacological, psychotherapeutic interventions becomes important. In this chapter, we have introduced various modalities of psychotherapy and provided evidence and indications for each based on the presenting diagnosis. Various types of psychotherapy delivered in different settings have been approved for a number of psychiatric disorders and should be utilized as stand-alone or adjunctive therapies.

References

1. Christensen K, Doblhammer G, Rau R, Vaupel JW. Ageing populations: the challenges ahead. *Lancet*. 2009;374 (9696):1196–1208. doi: 10.1016/S0140-6736(09)61460-4

2. Jeste DV, Savla GN, Thompson WK, et al. Older age is associated with more successful aging: role of resilience and depression. *Am J Psychiatry*. 2013;170 (2):188–196. doi: 10.1176/appi. ajp.2012.12030386

3. Delle FA, Bassi M, Boccaletti ES, et al. Promoting well-being in old age: the psychological benefits of two training programs of adapted physical activity. *Front Psychol*. 2018;9:828. doi: 10.3389/fpsyg.2018.00828

4. Hollon SD, DeRubeis RJ, Shelton RC, et al. Prevention of relapse following cognitive therapy vs medications in moderate to severe depression. *Arch Gen Psychiatry*. 2005;62(4): 417–422.

5. Thompson LW, Coon DW, Gallagher-Thompson D, Sommer BR, Koin D. Comparison of desipramine and cognitive/behavioral therapy in the treatment of elderly outpatients with mild-to-moderate

depression. *Am J Geriatr Psychiatry.* 2001;9(3):225–240.

6. Alexopoulos GS, Raue PJ, Gunning F, et al. "Engage" therapy: behavioral activation and improvement of late-life major depression. *Am J Geriatr Psychiatry.* 2016;24(4):320–326. doi: 10.1016/j.jagp.2015.11.006

7. Tavares LR, Barbosa MR. Efficacy of group psychotherapy for geriatric depression: a systematic review. *Arch Gerontol Geriatr.* 2018;78:71–80. doi: 10.1016/j.archger.2018.06.001

8. Liu B, Tan Y, Cai D, et al. A study of the clinical effect and dropout rate of drugs combined with group integrated psychotherapy on elderly patients with depression. *Shanghai Arch Psychiatry.* 2018;30(1):39–46. doi: 10.11919/j.issn.1002-0829.217051

9. DeRubeis RJ, Hollon SD, Amsterdam JD, et al. Cognitive therapy vs medications in the treatment of moderate to severe depression. *Arch Gen Psychiatry.* 2005;62:409–415.

10. Rush AJ, Beck AT, Kovacs M, Hollon S. Comparative efficacy of cognitive therapy and pharmacotherapy in the treatment of depressed patients. *Cognit Ther Res.* 1977;1:17–37.

11. Jacobson NS, Hollon SD. Cognitive-behavior therapy versus pharmacotherapy: now that the jury's returned its verdict, it's time to present the rest of the evidence. *J Consult Clin Psychol.* 1996;64:74–80.

12. Hollon SD, DeRubeis RJ, Evans MD, et al. Cognitive therapy and pharmacotherapy for depression: singly and in combination. *Arch Gen Psychiatry.* 1992;49:774–781.

13. Hobbs MJ, Joubert AE, Mahoney AEJ, Andrews G. Treating late-life depression: comparing the effects of internet-delivered cognitive behavior therapy across the adult lifespan. *J Affect Disord.* 2018;226:58–65. doi: 10.1016/j.jad.2017.09.026

14. Egede LE, Acierno R, Knapp RG, et al. Psychotherapy for depression in older veterans via telemedicine: a randomised, open-label, non-inferiority trial. *Lancet Psychiatry.* 2015;2(8):693–701. doi: 10.1016/S2215-0366(15)00122-4

15. Moral JCM, Terrero FBF, Galán AS, Rodríguez TM. Effect of integrative reminiscence therapy on depression, well-being, integrity, self-esteem, and life satisfaction in older adults. *J Posit Psychol.* 2015;10(3):240–247.

16. Wu LF. Group integrative reminiscence therapy on self-esteem, life satisfaction and depressive symptoms in institutionalized older veterans. *J Clin Nurs.* 2011 Aug;20(15–16):2195–2203. doi: 10.1111/j.1365-2702.2011.03699.x

17. Hsieh HF, Wang JJ. Effect of reminiscence therapy on depression in older adults: a systematic review. *Int J Nurs Stud.* 2003;40(4):335–345.

18. Watt LM, Cappeliez P. Integrative and instrumental reminiscence therapies for depression in older adults: intervention strategies and treatment effectiveness. *Aging Ment Health.* 2000;4(2):166–177.

19. Duewarke AR, Bridges AJ. Suicide interventions in primary care: a selective review of the evidence. *Fam Syst Health.* 2018;36(3):289–302. doi:10.1037/fsh0000349

20. Thompson LW, Gallagher D. Efficacy of psychotherapy in the treatment of late-life depression. *Adv Behav Res Ther.* 1984;6(2):127–139.

21. Alexopoulos GS, Raue P, Areán P. Problem-solving therapy versus supportive therapy in geriatric major depression with executive dysfunction. *Am J Geriatric Psychiatry.* 2003;11(1):46–52.

22. Gök Ugur H, Yaman Aktaş Y, Orak OS, Saglambilen O, Aydin Avci İ. The effect of music therapy on depression and physiological parameters in elderly people living in a Turkish nursing home: a randomized-controlled trial. *Aging Ment Health.* 2017;12(21):1280–1286.

23. McCaffrey R, Liehr P, Gregersen T, Nishioka R. Garden walking and art therapy for depression in older adults: a pilot study. *Res Gerontol Nurse.* 2011;4(4):237–242. doi: 10.3928/19404921-20110201-01

24. Laborde-Lahoz P, El-Gabalawy R, Kinley J, et al. Subsyndromal depression among older adults in the USA: prevalence, comorbidity, and risk for new-onset psychiatric disorders in late life. *Int J Geriatr Psychiatry*. 2015;30(7):677–685. doi: 10.1002/gps.4204

25. Vanltallie TB. Subsyndromal depression in the elderly: underdiagnosed and undertreated. *Metabolism*. 2005;54 (5):39–44.

26. Reynolds CF 3rd, Thomas SB, Morse JQ, et al. Early intervention to preempt major depression among older black and white adults. *Psychiatr Serv*. 2014;65(6):765–773. doi: 10.1176/appi.ps.201300216

27. Kasckow J, Klaus J, Morse J, et al. Using problem solving therapy to treat veterans with subsyndromal depression: a pilot study. *Int J Geriatr Psychiatry*. 2014;29 (12):1255–1261. doi: 10.1002/gps.4105

28. Rawtaer I, Mahendran R, Yu J, et al. Psychosocial interventions with art, music, Tai Chi and mindfulness for subsyndromal depression and anxiety in older adults: a naturalistic study in Singapore. *Asia Pac Psychiatry*. 2015;7(3):240–250. DOI: 10.1111/appy.12201

29. Ramos K, Stanley MA. Anxiety disorders in late life. *Psychiatr Clin North Am*. 2017;41 (1):55–64. doi: 10.1016/j.psc.2017.10.005

30. Leipzig RM, Cumming RG, Tinetti ME. Drugs and falls in older people: a systematic review and meta-analysis: II. Cardiac and analgesic drugs. *J Am Geriatri Soc*. 1999;47(1):40–50.

31. Gould RL, Coulson MC, Howard RJ. Efficacy of cognitive behavioral therapy for anxiety disorders in older people: a meta-analysis and meta-regression of randomized controlled trials. *J Am Geriatr Soc*. 2012 Feb;60(2):218–229. doi: 10.1111/ j.1532-5415.2011.03824.x

32. Hall J, Kellett S, Berrios R, Bains MK, Scott S. Efficacy of cognitive behavioral therapy for generalized anxiety disorder in older adults: systematic review, meta-analysis, and meta-regression. *Am J Geriatr Psychiatry*. 2016 Nov 1;24 (11):1063–1073.

33. Hendriks GJ, Keijsers GP, Kampman M, et al. Treatment of anxiety disorders in the elderly. *Tijdschr Psychiatr*. 2011;53 (9):589–595.

34. Wetherell JL, Gatz M, Craske MG. Treatment of generalized anxiety disorder in older adults. *J Consult Clin Psychol*. 2003;71(1):31–40.

35. Ayers CR, Sorrell JT, Thorp SR, Wetherell JL. Evidence-based psychological treatments for late-life anxiety. *Psychol Aging*. 2007;22(1):8–17.

36. Thorp SR, Ayers CR, Nuevo R, et al. Meta-analysis comparing different behavioral treatments for late-life anxiety. *Am J Geriatr Psychiatry*. 2009;17(2):105–115. doi: 10.1097/JGP.0b013e31818b3f7e

37. Wetherell JL, Afari N, Ayers CR, et al. Acceptance and commitment therapy for generalized anxiety disorder in older adults: a preliminary report. *Behav Ther*. 2011;42 (1):127–134. doi: 10.1016/j. beth.2010.07.002

38. Hazlett-Stevens H, Singer J, Chong A. Mindfulness-based stress reduction and mindfulness-based cognitive therapy with older adults: a qualitative review of randomized controlled outcome research. *Clinical Gerontologist*. 2018 Sep 13;42(4): 347–358.

39. Rybarczyk B, Stepanski E, Fogg L, et al. A placebo-controlled test of cognitive-behavioral therapy for comorbid insomnia in older adults. *J Consult Clin Psychol*. 2005;73(6):1164–1174.

40. Morin CM, Kowatch RA, Barry T, Walton E. Cognitive-behavior therapy for late-life insomnia. *J Consult Clin Psychol*. 1993;61 (1):137–146.

41. Buysse DJ, Germain A, Moul DE, et al. Efficacy of brief behavioral treatment for chronic insomnia in older adults. *Arch Intern Med*. 2011;171(10):887–895. doi: 10.1001/archinternmed.2010.535

42. Amad A, Geoffroy PA, Vaiva G, Thomas P. Personality and personality disorders in the elderly: diagnostic, course and management. *Encephale*. 2013;39 (5):374–382. doi: 10.1016/j. encep.2012.08.006

43. Lynch TR, Cheavens JS, Cukrowicz KC, et al. Treatment of older adults with co-morbid personality disorder and depression: a dialectical behavior therapy approach. *Int J Geriatr Psychiatry*. 2007;22 (2):131–143.

44. Videler AC, van Alphen SPJ, van Royen RJJ, et al. Schema therapy for personality disorders in older adults: a multiple-baseline study. *Aging Ment Health*. 2018;22 (6):738–747. doi: 10.1080/ 13607863.2017.1318260

45. Liang JH, Xu Y, Lin L, et al. Comparison of multiple interventions for older adults with Alzheimer disease or mild cognitive impairment: a PRISMA-compliant network meta-analysis. *Medicine (Baltimore)*. 2018;97(20):e10744. doi: 10.1097/ MD.0000000000010744

46. Joosten-Weyn Banningh LW, Prins JB, Vernooij-Dassen MJ, et al. Group therapy for patients with mild cognitive impairment and their significant others: results of a waiting-list controlled trial. *Gerontology*. 2011;57(5):444–454. doi: 10.1159/000315933

47. Cheston R. Psychotherapeutic work with people with dementia: a review of the literature. *Br J Med Psychol*. 1998;71 (3):211–231.

48. Douglas S, James I, Ballard C. Non-pharmacological interventions in dementia. *Adv Psychiatric Treat*. 2004 May;10 (3):171–177.

49. Rabins PV. Developing treatment guidelines for Alzheimer's disease and other dementias. *J Clin Psychiatry*. 1996;57:37–38.

50. Woods B, Spector A, Jones C, Orrell M, Davies S. Reminiscence therapy for dementia. *Cochrane Database of Syst Rev*. 2005;18(2):203–205.

51. Gum A, Areán PA. Current status of psychotherapy for mental disorders in the elderly. *Curr Psychiatry Rep*. 2004;6 (1):32–38.

52. Hund B, Reuter K, Harter M, et al. Stressors, symptom profile, and predictors of adjustment disorder in cancer patients. Results from an epidemiological study with the composite internal diagnostic interview, adaptation for oncology (CIDI-O). *Depress Anxiety*. 2016;33(2):153–161. doi: 10.1002/da.22441

53. Mitchell AJ, Sheth B, Gill J, et al. Prevalence and predictors of post-stroke mood disorders: a meta-analysis and meta-regression of depression, anxiety, and adjustment disorder. *Gen Hosp Psychiatry*. 2017;47:48–60. doi: 10.1016/j. genhosppsych.2017.04.001

54. Haase M, Frommer J, Franke GH, et al. From symptom relief to interpersonal change: treatment outcome and effectiveness in inpatient psychiatry. *Psychother Res*. 2008;18(5):615–624. doi: 10.1080/10503300802192158

55. Hsiao FH, Lai YM, Chen YT, et al. Efficacy of psychotherapy on diurnal cortisol patterns and suicidal ideation in adjustment disorder with depressed mood. *Gen Hosp Psychiatry*. 2014;36(2):214–219. doi: 10.1016/j.genhosppsych.2013.10.019

56. Sundquist J, Lilja A, Palmer K, et al. Mindfulness group therapy in primary care patients with depression, anxiety and stress and adjustment disorders: randomized controlled trial. *Br J Psychiatry*. 2015;206 (2):128–135. doi: 10.1192/bjp. bp.114.150243

57. Shimizu K, Akizuki N, Nakaya N, et al. Treatment response to psychiatric intervention and predictors of response among cancer patients with adjustment disorders. *J Pain Symptom Manage*. 2011;41(4):684–691. doi:10.1016/j. jpainsymman.2010.07.011

58. Shear MK, Wang Y, Skritskaya N, et al. Treatment of complicated grief in elderly persons: a randomized clinical trial. *JAMA Psychiatry*. 2014;71(11):1287–1295. doi: 10.1001/jamapsychiatry.2014.1242

59. Shear K. Complicated grief. *N Engl J Med*. 2015 Jan;372:153–160. doi: 10.1056/ NEJMcp1315618

60. Shear K, Frank E, Houck PR, Reynolds CF 3rd. Treatment of complicated grief: a randomized controlled trial. *JAMA*. 2005 Jun;293(21):2601–2608. doi:10.1001/ jama.293.21.2601

61. Shear MK, Reynolds CF 3rd, Simon NM, et al. Optimizing treatment of complicated grief: a randomized clinical trial. *JAMA Psychiatry.* 2016;73(7):685–694. doi: 10.1001/jamapsychiatry.2016.0892

62. Ehde DM, Dillworth TM, Turner JA. Cognitive-behavioral therapy for individuals with chronic pain: efficacy, innovations, and directions for research. *Am Psychol.* 2014;69(2):153–166. doi: 10.1037/a0035747

63. Gatchel RJ, Peng YB, Peters ML, Fuchs PN, Turk DC. The biopsychosocial approach to chronic pain: scientific advances and future directions. *Psychol Bull.* 2007;133 (4):581–624. doi:10.1037/0033-2909.133.4.581

64. Mattenklodt P, Leonhardt C. Psychological assessment and psychotherapy for chronic pain in the elderly. *Schmerz.* 2015 Aug;29 (4):349–361. doi: 10.1007/s00482-015-0007-3

65. Nicholas MK, Asghari A, Blyth FM, et al. Self-management intervention for chronic pain in older adults: a randomized controlled trial. *Pain.* 2013;154:824–835. doi:10.1016/j.pain.2013.02.009

66. Yi JL, Porucznik CA, Gren LH, et al. The impact of preoperative mindfulness-based stress reduction on postoperative patient-reported pain, disability, quality of life, and prescription opioid use in lumbar spine degenerative disease: a pilot study. *World Neurosurg.* 2019;121:e786–e791. doi: 10.1016/j.wneu.2018.09.223

67. Morone NE, Greco CM, Moore CG, et al. A mind-body program for older adults with chronic lower back pain: a randomized clinical trial. *JAMA Intern Med.* 2016 Mar;176(3):329–337. doi: 10.1001/jamainternmed.2015.8033

68. Blanchard EB, Appelbaum KA, Radnitz CL, et al. A controlled evaluation of thermal biofeedback and thermal biofeedback combined with cognitive therapy in treatment of vascular headache. *J Consult Clin Psychol.* 1990 Apr;58(2):216–224.

69. Gfroerer J, Penne M, Pemberton M, Folsom R. Substance abuse treatment need among older adults in 2020: the impact of the aging baby-boom cohort. *Drug Alcohol Depend.* 2003 Mar;69(2):127–135.

70. United States Department of Health and Human Services. Substance Abuse and Mental Health Services Administration. Center for Behavioral Health Statistics and Quality. National survey on drug use and health. 2017 [cited 2018 Dec 28]. Retrieved from: www.samhsa.gov/data/nsduh/reports-detailed-tables-2017-NSDUH

71. Fleming MF, Manwell LB, Barry KL, Adams W, Stauffacher EA. Brief physician advice for alcohol problems in older adults: a randomized community-based trial. *J Fam Pract.* 1999 May;48(5):378–384.

72. Gordon AJ, Conigliaro J, Maisto SA, et al. Comparison of consumption effects of brief interventions for hazardous drinking elderly. *Subst Use Misuse.* 2003 Jan;38 (8):1017–1035.

73. Outlaw FH, Marquart JM, Roy A, et al. Treatment outcomes for older adults who abuse substances. *J Appl Gerontol.* 2012 Feb;31(1):78–100.

74. Slaymaker VJ, Owen P. Alcohol and other drug dependence severity among older adults in treatment: measuring characteristics and outcomes. *Alcoholism Treat Q.* 2008 Jun;26(3):259–273.

75. Oslin DW, Pettinati H, Volpicelli JR. Alcoholism treatment adherence: older age predicts better adherence and drinking outcomes. *Am J Geriatr Psychiatry.* 2002 Nov;10(6):740–747.

76. Sorocco KH, Ferrell SW. Alcohol use among older adults. *J Gen Psychol.* 2006 Oct;133(4):453–467.

77. Barrick C, Connors GJ. Relapse prevention and maintaining abstinence in older adults with alcohol-use disorders. *Drugs Aging.* 2002 Aug;19(8):583–594.

78. Steptoe A., Deaton A., Stone A. Psychological wellbeing, health and ageing. *Lancet.* 2015;385(9968):640–648. doi: 10.1016/S0140-6736(13)61489-0

79. Jeste DV and Palmer BW. A call for a new positive psychiatry of ageing. *Br J Psychiatry.* 2013;202:81–83. doi: 10.1192/bjp.bp.112.110643

80. Marquine MJ, Zlatar ZZ, Sewell DD. Positive geriatric and cultural psychiatry. In: Jeste DV, Palmer BW, editors. *Positive psychiatry*. Arlington, VA: American Psychiatric Publishing; 2015. p. 305–324.

81. Preschl B, Maercker A, Wagner B, et al. Life-review therapy with computer supplements for depression in the elderly: a randomized controlled trial. *Aging Ment Health*. 2012;16(8):964–974. doi: 10.1080/13607863.2012.702726

82. Frieswijk N, Steverink N, Buunk BP, Slaets JPJ. The effectiveness of a bibliotherapy in increasing the self-management ability of slightly to moderately frail older people. *Patient Educ Couns*. 2006;61(2):219–227.

83. D'Zurilla TJ, Nezu AM. *Problem-solving therapy: a social competence approach to clinical intervention*. 2nd ed. New York: Springer; 1999.

84. Nezu AM, Maguth Nezu C, D'Zurilla TJ. *Problem-solving therapy: a treatment manual*. New York: Springer; 2013.

85. Kropf N, Cummings S. Problem-solving therapy: theory and practice. In: *Evidence-based treatment and practice with older adults: theory, practice, and research*.

Oxford: Oxford University Press; 2017. p. 87–102.

86. Brodie DA, Inoue A, Shaw DG. Motivational interviewing to change quality of life for people with chronic heart failure: a randomised controlled trial. *Int J Nurs Stud*. 2008;45(4):489–500.

87. Kang HY, Gu MO. Development and effects of a motivational interviewing self-management program for elderly patients with diabetes mellitus. *J Korean Acad Nurs*. 2015;45(4):533–543. doi: 10.4040/jkan.2015.45.4.533

88. Burke BL, Arkowitz H, Menchola M. The efficacy of motivational interviewing: a meta-analysis of controlled clinical trials. *J Consult Clin Psychol*. 2003;71(5):843–861.

89. Heisel M, Talbot NL, King DA, Tu XM, Duberstein PR. Adapting interpersonal psychotherapy for older adults at risk for suicide. *Am J Geriatr Psychiatry*. 2015;23(1):87–98. doi: 10.1016/j.jagp.2014.03.010

90. Sutipan P, Intarakamhang U, Macaskill A. The impact of positive psychological interventions on well-being in healthy elderly people. *J Happiness Stud*. 2017;18(1):269–91.

Choice of Psychotherapy Approach

Feyza Marouf

Introduction

Barriers to Referral

More than 15% of elderly Americans struggle with mental illness, yet only 3% seek mental health care.[1,2] Middle class, partnered minorities with mild symptoms, including those individuals without cognitive decline, are the least likely to pursue mental health services, especially those living in rural areas.[3] The vast underutilization of psychotherapy in late life can be understood in part due to the individual's reluctance to engage in treatment, including the discomfort of interacting with mental health professionals and the belief that symptoms may improve on their own.[4] Members of the "Silent Generation" (those born between 1925 and 1945) are generally unfamiliar with psychotherapy as a treatment option or as an adjunct to medication management. They may interpret mood and anxiety symptoms as signs of physical rather than mental illness, or worry that disclosure of psychiatric distress could lead to involuntary hospitalization or placement outside the home.[5]

Misconceptions about the role of psychotherapy in late life also extend to healthcare providers. Mental illness among older adults is most frequently diagnosed in primary care settings, and elderly patients usually defer to their physicians for treatment recommendations.[6] The complexity of needs in late life, including adapting to and coping with medical illness, physical limitations and cognitive changes, can lead to prioritization of physical over mental health.[8] Although older adults indicate a preference for psychotherapy when compared to other treatment approaches, most depressed and anxious elders are usually prescribed medications, sometimes at rates higher than in the younger population.[9–11] Provider beliefs that depression and anxiety are a natural part of aging, in addition to uncertainty about the effectiveness of psychotherapy among older adults, can interfere with appropriate referrals. Even among primary care physicians with positive opinions of psychotherapy, only one in four prescribes psychotherapy alone for mild to moderate late-life depression.[7] Limited access and availability of gero-psychologists, as well as reimbursement constraints create further barriers to treatment.

Choosing a Therapeutic Modality

Despite low utilization rates, psychotherapy is a very effective treatment in late life. Cognitive behavioral therapy (CBT), interpersonal psychotherapy (IPT), problem-solving therapy (PST), and brief dynamic psychotherapy (BDP) have all been used with success in the geriatric population.[12,13] Cognitive therapies have the strongest evidence base for depression and anxiety, especially in the setting of medical illness.[14,15] Problem-solving

23

therapies offer a behavioral approach that can be particularly effective for executive dysfunction.[16] Interpersonal therapies are readily applicable to older adults struggling with complicated grief, retirement, or family conflict.[17] Brief psychodynamic treatment can be particularly useful for patients with mild to moderate depression struggling with self-esteem or acceptance of mortality.

The sense of limited time remaining in their lives can accelerate the wish for psychological change among older adults. Although rarely surprised by feelings of sadness, emptiness, and loneliness as they age, most older adults do not anticipate the irritability, anger, fatigue, and insomnia that can occur in the setting of increased dependency, debility, and loss. Actual losses frequently exist alongside fears of future losses, including the loss of possibilities.[18] To make the most use of psychotherapy, older adults must be willing to accept help. This can be especially challenging for members of the Silent Generation, a stoic cohort who emphasize personal responsibility, prefer not to depend on others, and can be reluctant to express or discuss their emotions.[19] Baby Boomers, in comparison, are frequently more familiar with the process and benefits of psychotherapy.[20]

Deciding on the best course of psychotherapy for an older adult begins with a comprehensive case formulation. Noting an individual's coping style, doubts, level of self-criticism, and unresolved resentments can guide the goals of treatment. Medical workup and neuropsychological testing help clarify the impact of illness on patient adaptation. Understanding the patient's capacity to tolerate affect, lead a session, and sit with silence helps a provider decide between more structured therapies like CBT or PST and less directive, affect-focused modalities like IPT or brief dynamic psychotherapy. Newer caregivers, for example, show a preference for expressive, psychodynamic treatments compared to long-term caregivers, who may engage best with a problem-solving approach.[21]

For the debilitated older adult, lack of energy due to medical conditions can combine with helplessness and lead to the abandonment of care. Individuals with weaker social networks face the most difficulty. Evaluation of physical and functional limitations helps determine the most appropriate treatment setting for these individuals. Shorter psychotherapies like PST can be particularly useful with severely medically ill adults, as can inhome therapies like self-guided cognitive behavioral therapy. Therapies that can be easily delivered in primary care settings, like CBT, PST, and IPT are effective in this setting, even when the interval between sessions extends to two weeks.[22–24] While normal age-related changes in cognition do not usually interfere with the delivery or effectiveness of psychotherapy, more marked impairments can complicate treatment. Memory impairments and cognitive slowing can particularly affect the success of learning-based therapies, including CBT and problem-solving therapy.[25]

Older adults represent a very diverse group of individuals. Adaptations to psychotherapy, including briefer sessions, repetition, and shortening treatment length should be based on individual needs and not age. Some older adults bring with them a history of positive relationships, strong coping strategies, and resilience to injury. Others may have experienced deep distress in addition to positive moments. Still others may be struggling with severe mood or personality disorders (PDs) that make basic attachment difficult. Indeed, older adults tend to decide quickly if a therapist is trustworthy, has the necessary expertise to address the individual's concerns, and will take the time to understand them.[26] More elderly individuals terminate therapy after the initial visit than at any other point in treatment.[27] The relationship between individuals and their therapists is critical for psychotherapy to be effective, regardless of the theoretical approach.[28]

Common Factors

Therapy provides a space, sometimes for the first time, where older adults can safely discuss their difficulties. On average, elderly individuals make excellent use of psychotherapy, confronting difficult material in the pursuit of intra-psychic, interpersonal, and behavioral change. Factors common to all psychotherapies, including empathy, alliance, positive regard, and expectations, may account for much of the variability in psychotherapy outcomes.[29–31] Therapist skills and techniques, including exploration, reflection, and accurate interpretation, in addition to a flexible and honest approach, all contribute to the formation of a positive relationship.[32]

Positive client perception of the therapeutic relationship is associated with a reduction in symptoms and increased treatment efficacy.[33] Feelings of understanding and acceptance promote social connection and contribute to favorable patient expectations, while warm, respectful and empathic engagement strengthens the therapeutic bond.[34] This may be truer with motivated and cooperative individuals than among individuals with interpersonal difficulties, although the impact of therapist skills when compared to client characteristics has yet to be sufficiently examined. However, research suggests that the most effective therapists are able to form alliances across a range of clients.[35]

Early in treatment, psychotherapists discuss with their clients the tasks and goals at hand. Discussion and agreement are critical components of the therapeutic alliance.[36,37] Careful review of expectations, including an explanation of the limits of therapy, steers the course of therapy forward. Older adults often enter psychotherapy with their own explanations of illness, heavily influenced by cultural conceptualizations. Treatments that can be adapted to be congruent with cultural beliefs are more likely to be effective than unadapted evidence-based treatments.[38]

Understanding and accepting the rationale for treatment is necessary for individuals to build confidence about the possibilities of treatment outcome. A strong alliance reinforces the belief that participating in treatment will lead to better coping with difficulties. Research on expectations correlates the individual's ratings with treatment outcomes, but most studies measure these expectations prior to the therapist's explanation of treatment. The relationship between expectations and outcome may be relatively small, although still statistically significant.[39]

Specific Therapies

Cognitive Behavioral Therapy

Most therapists who emphasize the importance of common factors in the treatment of psychiatric illness also concede that specific techniques, so-called special ingredients, can be particularly effective for certain conditions. For example, CBT is quite successful in the management of phobic anxiety, even more effective among older adults when compared to younger individuals.[42] As an explicit, theory-driven approach, CBT is highly structured and manualized to facilitate training and delivery of treatment. Cognitive behavioral therapy works effectively for both depression and anxiety in late life, and has become a model of evidence-based treatment, although researcher allegiance and weak comparators limit the evidence base.[43,44] While a strong working relationship between the client and the therapist is necessary for CBT, the relationship alone is not sufficient to ensure good treatment outcomes.[45]

Cognitive behavioral therapy assumes that maladaptive patterns of thought and behavior contribute to the development of emotional distress. Close appraisal of an individual's experience of an event, rather than the event itself, is a key ingredient in therapeutic change. Cognitive behavioral therapists tend to be clear, open and direct, which can be particularly reassuring for older adults. By emphasizing skill building in a present-oriented, problem-focused way, CBT promotes self-agency. This can be particularly important for older adults who endorse strong cohort beliefs about independence and personal responsibility.

Cognitive behavioral therapy works as well for depressed older adults as it does for the younger population, although most of this data does not include the oldest-old.[46] For depressed older adults with mild cognitive impairment (CI) and various medical conditions – from falls and fractures to chronic obstructive pulmonary disease (COPD) to heart disease and neurological illness – CBT remains an effective treatment.[47–49] Approximately 80% of individuals with depression and Parkinson's disease were able to complete an 8-week course of CBT that resulted in a decrease in depression severity and fewer hospitalizations after the intervention.[50]

Cognitive behavioral therapy is also useful across a range of late-life anxiety disorders, including generalized anxiety disorder (GAD), panic disorder, and mixed anxiety disorders, with effect sizes comparable to that those in younger adults. Older adults may have an advantage over younger adults in reducing avoidance behaviors through cognitive behavioral therapy.[51] For treatments delivered in primary care, two large randomized clinical trials demonstrated the effectiveness of CBT for late-life generalized anxiety disorder. In both trials, treatment included a combination of skills-based sessions and follow-up booster calls.[52] When compared with treatment as usual (TAU), control, or waitlist conditions, CBT was clearly a superior choice for the treatment of anxiety.[53] However, when compared with supportive therapy, treatment differences appeared more modest.[54]

Increasingly, CBT is used in flexible delivery formats. Telephone-based CBT (CBT-T) for example, was more effective than an information-only control condition in reducing depression and worry among older adults with generalized anxiety disorder.[55] These benefits persisted up to a year after treatment completion.[56] Internet-based CBT may improve access to treatment as well as treatment engagement.[57] Further expansion of services may come from developing a broader workforce of mental health providers, including bachelor's degree-level mental health workers. Lay providers delivering CBT to anxious older adults in person and by telephone were found to have treatment outcomes comparable to PhD-level providers.[58]

Problem-Solving Therapy

Problem-solving therapy is a behavioral intervention targeting executive deficits in older adults with major depression that can result in significant improvements in depression, disability, cognitive impairment (CI), and also suicidal ideation (SI).[59] Problem-solving therapy focuses treatment on everyday problems and is brief, usually spanning six sessions. Patients are asked to identify problems including difficult thoughts, feelings, and interpersonal situations; assess the circumstances surrounding each problem; assign problems with low probability of change to lesser priority; and formulate feasible action plans for their top problems.[60] The goal of treatment is kept purposefully narrow, and patients are reminded that additional problems might fall beyond the scope of the therapy. Overall, PST stresses specific and realistic solutions.

Meta-analyses show that PST effectively treats late-life depression and can be more effective than other psychotherapies.[61,62] Studies evaluating treatment for depression in patients with CI frequently utilize problem-solving approaches and have concluded that PST results in significant improvement in measures of both depression and disability. In a multisite clinical trial of older adults with depression and executive dysfunction, PST was shown to be more effective than supportive therapy in reducing depressive symptoms, persisting long after the 12 weeks of treatment.[63] In a group of individuals undergoing stroke rehabilitation, the addition of PST resulted in significant improvements in task-oriented coping, decreased avoidance, and improved general quality of life when compared to treatment as usual.[64] Problem-solving therapy also has the potential to be an effective intervention for suicide by helping older adults reduce the potential for impulsive action and providing these individuals with the means for engaging in effective and risk-sensitive decision-making.[65]

Modified problem-solving treatments including primary care-based treatment, problem adaptation therapy (PATH), and homebound PST for individuals with cognitive impairment have also been effective in late-life depression.[66] Problem adaptation therapy is a home-delivered intervention that uses PST as a basic framework and incorporates environmental adaptations such as cues, reminders, timers, and step-by-step breakdown of tasks. Problem adaptation therapy also encourages family or caregiver participation to assist in problem-solving efforts and task completion. In a randomized controlled trial (RCT), PATH reduced depression severity and disability in comparison to supportive psychotherapy for the entire sample and reduced depression severity for the subgroup of individuals with mild to moderate dementia.[67]

Interpersonal Psychotherapy

Interpersonal psychotherapy is a less directive form of treatment than either CBT or PST and takes place over a longer course, usually 12–20 weekly sessions. Interpersonal psychotherapy focuses on targeting and resolving specific problems such as bereavement, role transitions, role disputes, or interpersonal conflicts.[68] These types of problems commonly occur among older adults, presenting as complicated grief, difficulty coping with retirement, marital conflicts, or difficulty accepting care, and can precipitate or worsen social isolation and loneliness, generating strong emotions that are difficult to tolerate, understand, and express. Miller and Silberman found that 42% of a sample of older adults reported that in order to recover from their depressive episode, they needed to resolve interpersonal conflicts, most frequently with spouses, children, and siblings.[69]

Interpersonal psychotherapy helps individuals resolve a problem by altering the problem itself, changing the relationship to the problem, or both. This framework distinguishes IPT from other therapeutic approaches, which identify the problem within the individual. With IPT, the therapeutic relationship becomes an important transitional support, providing a safe connection during a difficult crisis. Interpersonal psychotherapy utilizes common factors such as hope and the expectation for change, and emphasizes affect rather than cognitions, as well as short-term goals rather than open-ended exploration. Interpersonal psychotherapy also avoids the traditional focus on problematic personality patterns or attachment style, which can demoralize individuals and risk invalidating their experience of injury and distress.[70]

Interpersonal psychotherapy uses specific therapeutic techniques from a variety of approaches, including psychodynamic, supportive, and behavioral therapy. Enhancing social support, decreasing stress, facilitating emotional processing, and improving interpersonal skills are also mechanisms of change in interpersonal psychotherapy.[71] In addition to its effectiveness as an intervention for late-life depression, IPT is trans-diagnostic, and can be useful even for individuals with mild cognitive impairment. Here, modifications usually involve the integration of the caregiver into the treatment process, recognizing the role transition caregivers undergo in parallel to the individual's changing functional level. Interpersonal psychotherapy for cognitive impairment (IPT-CI) frequently targets disputes that arise around issues of care.[72]

Brief Dynamic Psychotherapy

Psychodynamic psychotherapy is an interpersonal form of psychotherapy that is also an intra-psychic, rather than behavioral, intervention. It should be considered for mild to moderate depressions where the goals of treatment are increased insight and improved adjustment. Frequently, older adults present for psychotherapy with a concrete concern and underreported levels of distress. As the situation is gradually explored, more intense feelings can emerge in relation to difficulty coping with disappointments and narcissistic injuries, fears of death, and other existential questions.[73] These are common themes of late-life psychotherapy, which places the issue of tolerating loss at the center of the therapeutic process.

Erikson described the major psychological task of late life as balancing the despairs of dwindling time with a sense of life's integrity. Even for highly functioning older adults, negotiating this developmental juncture can be daunting. Psychotherapists play a critical role in identifying and confronting false hopes, facilitating mourning, maintaining realistic appraisals of the future, and allowing individuals to authentically balance the satisfying and dissatisfying aspects of their lives.[74,75] For individuals with sufficient ego strength, dynamic treatment can be useful in connecting an individual's current distress with earlier, unresolved periods of development when needs were not adequately met. For example, a depressive episode may not be triggered by medical illness per se, but by how the experience of the illness returns the individual to an earlier life stage of problematic dependence. In such a scenario, engaging the individual's past can be cathartic, allowing the individual to acknowledge and accept disappointments while also recognizing and holding on to the worthwhile aspects of life.

Whereas long-term psychodynamic psychotherapy hopes to produce sustainable character change and emotional maturation, BDP centers on coping with a particular time of crisis. The specificity of the goals, the active role of the therapist, and the expectation that the course of therapy will be short – all these features distinguish short-term from long-term psychodynamic treatment.[76] In BDP, the therapist keeps the process reality based, such that old conflicts can be reexperienced within a new context, leading to positive change. This helps the individual build a positive sense of self while avoiding excessive dependency. Most individuals in BDP achieve insight and successfully terminate care without requiring long-term treatment.[77]

Future Directions

Psychotherapy research has historically been focused on categorical diagnoses and treatment outcomes, with little understanding of the mechanisms of change. Although at least 100 comparative psychotherapy trials have been conducted in adults, the effectiveness of any particular therapy is still uncertain.[78] Head-to-head comparisons generally involve CBT and acute symptom reduction, rather than other approaches and longer term effects. Meta-analyses of psychotherapies find small differences among various types of treatment, but minimal differences between total treatment and treatment without one or more critical ingredients.[79,80]

Proponents of specific factors tend to emphasize the evidence from RCTs, despite the limitations of these trials. By and large, most evidence-based psychotherapies are delivered to discrete diagnostic groups in highly controlled and academic research settings. There-fore, the generalizability of outcomes remains unclear. Trials often favor internal rather than external validity, enrolling individuals with fewer comorbidities who rarely represent clients in real-world clinics.[81,82] Low-quality studies distort effect sizes, while negative trials are less likely to be reported. One systematic review revealed that only 12% of psychotherapy trials were prospectively registered with clearly defined primary outcome measures.[83]

For older adults, the psychotherapy evidence base is limited by the presence of only a small number of vastly underpowered studies.[54] Comparisons with waitlist controls may exaggerate the effects of cognitive therapy, given that comparisons to supportive therapy, perhaps the best control for common factors, are often much more modest. In the absence of process-focused studies, distinguishing whether the key aspects of successful treatments are related to common or specific factors remains exceedingly hard. For example, a therapist's rigid adherence to theory-specific factors may reduce alliance with an older adult, who then becomes more resistant to accepting treatment. In addition, client rejection of a particular therapeutic modality may reflect difficulties with the therapist's demeanor and empathy rather than the applicability of specific techniques.[84,85]

The therapeutic alliance is a dyadic construct, reflecting a reciprocal working relation-ship. By and large, emotions are processed and regulated in relational systems, rather than internally. This is quite different from the medical model of the individual as a recipient of the therapist's activities, which underlies most objective, cognitive, and behavioral treat-ments. Future research must better address the therapist as an independent variable in the setting of strong alliance effects. Neuroimaging studies also have the potential to expand our understanding of the pathways of psychotherapeutic change.[86] The development of internet-based virtual therapies offers an opportunity to determine which specific compon-ents of treatment are necessary for change to occur.[87]

Conclusion

Despite the preference of older adults for choosing psychotherapy over medication as a treatment modality, studies show low rates of psychotherapy use by older adults and few visits even when treatment is initiated. Older adults often present for psychotherapy with multiple losses, including bereavement, physical and cognitive decline, and reduc-tions of social supports. What can be achieved therapeutically depends on the individ-ual's ability to reconcile hope with the reality of despair. It is worth considering that most older adults have survived into old age despite significant adversities. Engaging with the individual experience of each older adult helps psychotherapists decide on the main presenting problems, the individual's capacity for different types of psychological work, and the applicability of various treatment modalities to the needs at hand. The importance of specific therapeutic ingredients relies on comparisons with plausible controls, whereas the impact of common therapeutic factors stems from correlations between therapy outcomes and individual reports of rapport and engagement. Deficits of the existing evidence base are related to the low power and small number of studies. To optimize treatment for older adults, research must better identify the specific mechanisms of therapeutic change.

References

1. CDC healthy aging data: the state of mental health and aging in America. Retrieved from: www.cdc.gov/aging/agingdata/data-portal/mental-health.html (May 10, 2019).

2. Byers AL, Arean PA, Yaffe K. Low use of mental health services among older Americans with mood and anxiety disorders. *Psychiatr Serv.* 2012;63(1):66–72.

3. Garrido MM, Kane RL, Kaas M, et al. Use of mental health care by community-dwelling older adults. *J Am Geriatr Soc.* 2011;59:50–56.

4. Karlin BE, Duffy M, Gleaves DH. Patterns and predictors of mental health service use and mental illness among older and younger adults in the United States. *Psychological Services.* 2008;5:275–294.

5. Mackenzie CS, Pagura J, Sareen J. Correlates of perceived need for and use of mental health services by older adults in the collaborative psychiatric epidemiology surveys. *Am J Geriatr Psychiatry.* 2010;18:1103–1115.

6. Wang PS, Lane M, Olfson M, et al. Twelve-month use of mental health services in the United States: results from the national comorbidity survey replication. *Arch Gen Psych.* 2005;62:629–640.

7. Verdoux H, Cortaredons S, Dumesnil H, Sebbah R, Verger P. Psychotherapy for depression in primary care: a panel survey of general practitioners' opinion and prescribing practice. *Social Psychiatry Psychiatr Epidemiol.* 2014;49:59–68.

8. Frost R, Beattie A, Bhanu C, Walters K, Ben-Shlomo Y. Management of epression and referral of over people to psychological therapies: a systematic review of qualitative studies. *Br J Gen Pract.* 2019;69(680):171–181.

9. Bosworth HB, Voils CI, Potter GG, Steffens DC. The effects of antidepressant medication adherence as well as psychosocial and clinical factors on depression outcome among older adults. *Int J Geriatr Psychiatry.* 2008;23(2):129–134.

10. Gum, A. M., Iser, L., Petkus, A. Behavioral health service utilization and preferences of older adults receiving home-based aging services. *Am J Geriatr Psychiatry.* 2010;18(6):491–501.

11. Olfson M, Marcus SC. National patterns in antidepressant medication treatment. *Arch Gen Psychiatry.* 2009;66(8):848–856.

12. Ayers CR, Sorrell JT, Thorp SR, Wetherell JL. Evidence-based psychological treatments for late life anxiety. *Psychol Aging.* 2007;22:8–17.

13. Samad Z, Brealey S, Gilbody S. The effectiveness of behavioral therapy for the treatment of depression in older adults. A meta-analysis. *Int J Geriatr Psychiatry.* 2011.

14. Laidlaw K, Davidson K, Toner H, et al. A randomized controlled trial of cognitive behavior therapy vs treatment as usual in the treatment of mild to moderate late life depression. *Int J Geriatr Psychiatry.* 2008;23(8):843–850.

15. Bower ES, Wetherell JL, Mon T, et al. Treating anxiety disorders in older adults: current treatments and future directions. *Harv Rev Psychiatry.* 2015;23:329–342.

16. Kiosses DN, Alexopoulos GS. Problem-solving therapy in the elderly. *Curr Treat Options Psychiatry.* 2014;1:15–26.

17. Lipsitz JD, Markowitz JC. Mechanisms of change in interpersonal therapy (IPT). *Clin Psychol Rev.* 2013;33(8):1134–1147.

18. Garner J. Psychotherapies and older adults. *Aust N Z J Psychiatry.* 2003;37:537–548.

19. Magai C, Cohen C, Milburn N, et al. Attachment styles in older European American and African American adults. *J Gerontol B Psychol Sci Soc Sci.* 2001;56 (10);S28–35.

20. O'Connor D, Kelson E. Boomer matters: responding to emotional health needs in an aging society. *J Gerontol Soc Work.* 2018;61 (1):61–77.

21. Gallagher-Thompson D, Steffen AM. Comparative effects of cognitive-behavioral and brief psychodynamic psychotherapies for depressed family caregivers. *J Consult Clin Psychol.* 1994;62:543–549.

22. Arean P, Hegel M, Vannoy S, et al. Effectiveness of problem-solving therapy for older, primary care patients with depression: results from the IMPACT project. *Gerontologist.* 2008;48:311–323.

23. Schulberg HC, Post EP, Raue PJ, et al. Treating late-life depression with interpersonal psychotherapy in the primary care sector. *Int J Geriatr Psychiatry.* 2007;22:106–114.

24. Gellis ZD, Bruce ML. Problem solving therapy for subthreshold depression in home healthcare patients with cardiovascular disease. *Am J Geriatr Psychiatry.* 2010;18:464–474.

25 Wilkins VM, Kiosses D, Ravdin LD. Late-life depression with comorbid cognitive impairment and disability: nonpharmacological interventions. *Clin Interv Aging.* 2010;5:323–331.

26. Willis J, Todorov A. First impressions: making up your mind after a 100-ms exposure to a face. *Psychol Sci.* 2006;17:592–598.

27. Connell J, Grant S, Mullin T. Client initiated termination of therapy at NHS primary care counselling services. *Couns Psychother Res.* 2006;6:60–7.

28. Markin R. Toward a common identity for relationally oriented clinicians: a place to hand one's hat. *Psychotherapy.* 2014;51:327–333.

29. Huppert JD, Fabbro A, Barlow DH. Evidence-based practice and psychological treatments. *Evidence-based psychotherapy:* where practice and research meet. 2006;131–152.

30. Crits-Christoph P, Gibbons MB, Hamilton J, Ring-Kurtz S, Gallop R. The dependability of alliance assessments: the alliance-outcome correlation is larger than you might think. *J Consult Clin Psychol.* 2011;79:267–278.

31. Wampold, BE, Flückiger, C, Del Re, AC, et al. In pursuit of truth: a critical examination of meta-analyses of cognitive behavior therapy. *Psychother Res.* 2017;27:14–32.

32. Arnow BA, Steidtmann D, Blasey C, et al. The relationship between the therapeutic alliance and treatment outcomes in two distinct therapies for chronic depression. *J Consult Clin Psychol.* 2013;81:627–638.

33. Mace RA, Gansler DA, Suvak MK, et al. Therapeutic relationship in the treatment of geriatric depression with executive dysfunction. *J Affect Disord.* 2017;214:130–137.

34. Ackerman SJ, Hilsenroth MJ. A review of therapist characteristics and techniques positively impacting the TA. *Clin Psychol Rev.* 2003;23:1–33.

35. Baldwin SA, Wampold BE, Imel ZE. Untangling the alliance-outcome correlation: exploring the relative importance of therapist and patient variability in the alliance. *J Consult Clin Psych.* 2007;75:842–852.

36. Crits-Christoph, P, Connolly Gibbons, MB, Crits-Christoph, K et al. Can therapists be trained to improve their alliances? A preliminary study of alliance-fostering psychotherapy. *Psychother Res.* 2006;16:268–281.

37. Horvath, AO. The alliance in context: accomplishments, challenges, and future directions. *Psychotherapy: Theory, Research, Practice, Training.* 2006;43:258–263.

38. Benish SG, Quintana S, Wampold BE. Culturally adapted psychotherapy and the legitimacy of myth: a direct-comparison meta-analysis. *J Couns Psychol.* 2011;58:279–289.

39. Constantino MJ, Arnkoff DB, Glass CR, et al. Expectations. *J Clin Psychol.* 2011;67:184–192.

40. Price DP, Finniss DG, Benedetti F. A comprehensive review of the placebo effect: recent advances and current thought. *Annu Rev Psychol.* 2008;59:565–590.

41. Benedetti, F. *Placebo effects: understanding the mechanisms in health and disease.* 2nd ed. New York: Oxford University Press; 2014.

42. Laidlaw K, Thompson LW, Dick-Siskin L, Gallagher-Thompson D. *Cognitive behaviour therapy with older people.* Chichester: John Wiley & Sons; 2003.

43. Pinquart M, Duberstein PR, Lyness JM. Treatments for later-life depressive conditions: a meta-analytic comparison of pharmacotherapy and CBT. *Am J Psychiatry.* 2006;163:1493–1501.

44. Wilson KC, Mottraam PG, Vassilas CA. Psychotherapeutic treatments for older depressed people. *Cochrane Database Syst Rev.* 2008 Jan 23;(1):CD004853.

45. Gould RL, Coulson MC, Howard RJ. Cognitive behavioral therapy for depression in older people: a meta-analysis and meta-regression of randomized controlled trials. *J Am Geriatr Soc.* 2012;60 (10):1817–1830.

46. Cuijpers P, Karyotaki E, Pot AM, et al. Managing depression in older age; psychological interventions. *Maturitas.* 2014; 79(2):160–169.

47. Joosten-Weyn Banningh LW, Kessels RP, lade Rikkert MG, et al. A cognitive behavioral group therapy for patients diagnosed with mild cognitive impairment and their significant others: feasibility and preliminary results. *Clin Rehabil.* 2008;22:731–740.

48. Freedland KE, Carney RM, Rich MW, et al. Cognitive behavior therapy for depression and self-care in heart failure patients: a randomized clinical trial. *JAMA Intern Med.* 2015;175:1773–1782.

49. Hummel J, Weisbrod C, Boesch L, et al. Acute illness and depression in elderly patients. Cognitive behavioral group psychotherapy in geriatric patients with comorbid depression: a randomized controlled trial. *JAMA.* 2017;18:341–349.

50. Calleo JS, Amspoker AB, Sarwar AI, et al. A pilot study of a cognitive-behavioral treatment for anxiety and depression in patients with Parkinson Disease. *J Geriatr Psychiatry Neurol.* 2015;28:210–217.

51. Hendriks G, Kampman M, Keijsers G, et al. Cognitive-behavioral therapy for panic disorder with agoraphobia in older adults: a comparison with younger patients. *Depress Anxiety.* 2014;31(8):669–677.

52. Stanley MA, Wilson N, Novy D, et al. Cognitive behavior therapy for generalized anxiety disorder among older adults in primary care. *J Am Med Assoc.* 2009;301 (14):1460–1467.

53. Thorp SR, Ayers C, Nuevo R, et al. Meta-analysis comparing different behavioral treatments for late-life anxiety. *Am J Geriatr Psychiatry.* 2009;17(2):105–115.

54. Huang AX, Delucchi K, Dunn LB et al. A systematic review and meta-analysis of psychotherapy for late-life depression. *Am J Geriatr Psychiatry.* 2015;233:261–273.

55. Brenes GA, Miller M, Williamson J, et al. A randomized controlled trial of telephone-delivered cognitive-behavioral therapy for late-life anxiety disorders. *Am J Geriatr Psychiatry.* 2012;20(8):707–716.

56. Brenes GA, Danhauer SC, Lyles MF, et al. Long term effects of telephone-delivered psychotherapy for late-life GAD. *Am J Geriatr Psychiatry.* 2017.

57. Staples LG, Fogliati VJ, Dear BF, Nielssen O, Titov N. Internet-delivered treatment for older adults with anxiety and depression: implementation of the Wellbeing Plus Course in routine clinical care and comparison with research trial outcomes. *BJPsych Open.* 2016;2(5):307–313.

58. Stanley MA, Wilson NL, Amspoker AB, et al. Lay providers can deliver effective cognitive behavior therapy for older adults with generalized anxiety disorder. *Depress Anxiety.* 2014;31(5):391–401.

59. Arean P, Hegel M, Vannoy S, et al. Effectiveness of problem-solving therapy for older, primary care patients with

depression: results from the IMPACT project. *Gerontologist.* 2008;48:311–323.

60. Choi NG, Marti CN, Conwell Y. Effect of problem-solving therapy on depressed low-income homebound older adults' death/suicidal ideation and hopelessness. *Suicide Life Threat Behav.* 2016;46:323–336.

61. Bell AC, Zurilla TJ. Problem solving therapy for depression: a meta-analysis. *Clin Psychol Rev.* 2009;29(4):348–353.

62. Malouff JM, Thorsteinsson EB, Schütte NS. The efficacy of problem solving therapy in reducing mental and physical health problems: a meta-analysis. *Clin Psychol Rev.* 2007;27(1):46–57.

63. Alexopoulos GS, Raue PJ, Kiosks DN, et al. Problem-solving therapy and supportive therapy in older adults with major depression and executive dysfunction: effect on disability. *Arch Gen Psychiatry.* 2011;68(1):33–41.

64. Visser MM, Heijenbrok-Kal MH, Van't Spijker A, et al. Problem-solving therapy during outpatient stroke rehabilitation improves coping and health-related quality of life: randomized controlled trials. *Stroke.* 2016;47(1):135–142.

65. Gustavson KA, Alexopoulos GS, Niu GC, et al. Problem-solving therapy reduces suicidal ideation in depressed older adults with executive dysfunction. *Am J Geriatr Psychiatry.* 2016;24(1):11–1766.

66. Arean PA, Raue P, Macken RS, et al. Problem-solving therapy and supportive therapy in older adults with major depression and executive dysfunction. *Am J Psychiatry.* 2010;167:1391–1398.

67. Kiosses DN, Ravdin LD, Gross JJ, et al. Problem adaptation therapy for older adults with major depression and cognitive impairment: a randomized clinical trial. *JAMA Psychiatry.* 2015;72(1):22–30.

68. Van Schaik A, van Marwijk H, Ader H, et al. Interpersonal psychotherapy for elderly patients in primary care. *Am J Geriatr Psychiatry.* 2006;14:777–786.

69. Markowitz JC, Milrod BL. The importance of responding to negative affect in psychotherapies. *Am J Psychiatry.* 2011;168(2):124–128.

70. Miller MD, Silberman RL. Using interpersonal psychotherapy with depressed elders. In: Zarit SH, Knight BG, editors. A guide to psychotherapy and aging: effective clinical interventions in a life-stage context. Washington, DC: American Psychological Association; 1996. p. 83–99.

71. Lipsitz JD, Markowitz JC. Mechanisms of change in interpersonal therapy (IPT). *Clin Psychol Rev.* 2013;33(8):1134–1147.

72. Miller MD, Reynolds CF 3rd. Expanding the usefulness of Interpersonal Psychotherapy (IPT) for depressed elders with co-morbid cognitive impairment. *Int J Geriatr Psychiatry.* 2007;22(2):101–105.

73. Morgan AC. Psychodynamic psychotherapy with older adults. *Psychiatric Services.* 2003;54(12):1592–1594.

74. Roseborough DJ, Luptak M, McLeod J, Bradshaw W. Effectiveness of psychodynamic psychotherapy with older adults: a longitudinal study. *Clinical Gerontologist.* 2012;36:1–16.

75. Nordhus I. Current psychodynamic approaches with older people. In: Laidlaw L, Knight B, editors. *Handbook of emotional disorders in later life.* New York: Oxford University Press; 2008. p. 165–182.

76. Kennedy GJ, Tanenbaum S. Psychotherapy with older adults. *Am J Psychotherapy.* 2000;54:386–407.

77. Critchley-Robbins S. Brief psychodynamic therapy with older people. In: Evans S, Garner J, editors. *Talking over the years: a handbook of dynamic psychotherapy with older adults.* New York: Brunner-Routledge; 2004.

78. Cuijpers P. Are all psychotherapies equally effective in the treatment of adult depression? The lack of statistical power of comparative outcome studies. *Evid Based Ment Health.* 2016;19:39–42.

79. Bell EC, Marcus DK, Goodlad JK. Are the parts as good as the whole? A meta-analysis of component treatment studies. *J Consult Clin Psychol.* 2013;81:722–736.

80. Ahn H, Wampold BE. Where oh where are the specific ingredients? A meta-analysis of

component studies in counseling and psychotherapy. *J Couns Psychol.* 2001;48:251–257.

81. Kaplan BJ, Giesbrecht G, Shannon S, McLeod K. Evaluating treatments in health care: the instability of a one-legged stool. *BMC Med Res Methodol.* 2011;11:65.

82. Rosenbaum P. The randomized controlled trial: an excellent design, but can it address the big questions in neurodisability? *Dev Med Child Neurol.* 2010; 52:111.

83. Bradley H, Rucklidge JJ, Mulder RT. A systematic review of trial registration and selective outcome reporting psychotherapy randomized controlled trials. *Acta Psychiatr Scand.* 2017;135:65–77.

84. Webb CA, DeRubeis RJ, Barber JP. Therapist adherence/competence and treatment outcome: a meta-analytic review. *J Consult Clin Psychol.* 2010;78: 200–211.

85. Owen J, Hilsenroth MJ. Treatment adherence: the importance of therapist flexibility in relation to therapy outcomes. *J Couns Psychol.* 2014;61: 280–288.

86. Fournier JC, Price RB. Psychotherapy and neuroimaging. *Focus* 2014;12: 290–298.

87. Mulder R, Murray G, Rucklidge J. Common versus specific factors in psychotherapy: opening the black box. *The Lancet Psychiatry.* 2017;4(12):953–962.

Chapter

4

Cognitive Behavioral Therapy in Late Life

Patricia Bamonti and M. Lindsey Jacobs

Introduction

Cognitive behavioral therapy (CBT) is a time-limited, collaborative, present-focused, skills-based intervention that focuses on behavioral and cognitive change in order to treat mental health conditions. The number of sessions is variable, although older adults typically require 16–20 sessions when treating mood or anxiety disorders.[1] Cognitive behavioral therapy is unique from other approaches in that it emphasizes active discovery and empirical examination of clients' interpretations, assumptions, and appraisals of the world. Cognitive behavioral therapy involves in-session and out-of-session practice for skill acquisition and generalization. Clients engage with therapeutic content through paper-and-pencil assignments, Socratic dialogue, role-plays, modeling, and behavioral experiments, with the goal of providing the client a set of cognitive and behavioral coping skills to use when faced with life stressors.

Cognitive behavioral therapy does not necessarily require modifications when working with cognitively intact older adults.[2] When modifications are made, they are used to optimize therapy by addressing deficits in cognition and sensory processing. Modifications may include adjusting the pace, using multiple modalities ("Say it, write it, show it"), interruption and redirection, repetition, and adjustment for sensory decline (large print, use of hearing aids, pocket talkers, magnifying glasses, digital recorders for sessions and homework).[3] Researchers have also emphasized the need for conceptual modifications, such as incorporating age-related developmental processes and the strengths and challenges that characterize late life.[4] Considering age-related developmental processes enhances treatment for many older adult patients and is akin to incorporating age-related developmental processes in earlier years of life (e.g., CBT with adolescents). When cognitive impairment (CI) or dementia is present, skills tend to focus on behavioral tasks with caregiver involvement.

Theoretical Framework

Cognitive behavioral therapy was developed based on the integration of two theories of psychopathology: cognitive[5] and behavioral.[6] Fundamental to CBT is the formulation that suffering is not directly caused by events themselves but is a result of clients' interpretation, appraisal, meaning, and behavioral response attached to events. Individuals' interpretation of the world occurs through schemas, which can be adaptive or maladaptive in nature.[7] In the case of depression, the negative cognitive triad is prominent, whereby beliefs are dominated by negative cognitions about oneself, others, and the world.[8] In anxiety, thinking is biased toward threat and danger and an underestimation of personal coping resources.[7]

Core beliefs, a type of schematic content, are central to the CBT model and refer to rigidly and overgeneralized beliefs about the self, others, and the world (e.g., "I am weak"). Intermediary beliefs are rules, assumptions, and attitudes individuals use to guide their lives (e.g., "I should do things myself"). Conditional rules are a specific type of intermediary belief and are readily identified because they usually take the form of an "If… then" statement (e.g., "If I open up to others, I will be rejected").[7] Individuals also engage in unhelpful coping behaviors, termed compensatory strategies, which are developed in response to core beliefs (e.g., avoidance). Finally, negative automatic thoughts (NATs) are the most obvious manifestation of maladaptive schemas and are characterized by automatic thoughts and images tied to a specific event (e.g., "I always mess up").

Behavior therapy (BT) is a core component of CBT based on the behavioral model of depression describing the connection between activity level and mood. The behavioral model posits that depressed mood results from a low rate of positive reinforcement and repeated exposure to aversive events.[6] The integrated cognitive-behavior model recognizes the role of cognition and behavior in precipitating and perpetuating distress. The CBT therapist focuses on the client's appraisal and interpretation of situations, as well as behaviors, such as avoidance, low rate of pleasant events, and skill deficits (e.g., problem-solving skills) that maintain psychological disorders.

Research Overview

Treatment effectiveness has been most widely researched in older adults with mood and anxiety disorders. Cognitive behavioral therapy is superior to waitlist controls and treatment as usual (TAU) for the treatment of depression.[9] Large effect sizes have been found for CBT,[10] and meta-analyses of controlled trial studies have shown CBT to be equally as effective as reminiscence therapy (RT) at reducing depressive symptoms in older adults.[10,11] Research comparing CBT to other psychotherapies has found CBT to be equally or more effective compared to other treatments.[9,10,12] A meta-analysis of 23 randomized controlled trials (RCTs) published between 1982 and 2009 found that CBT was equally effective compared to other treatments.[9] In contrast, another meta-analysis that compared the effects of 26 controlled intervention studies published between 1982 and 2006 found that CBT was more effective than psychodynamic therapy, BT, cognitive therapy, interpersonal psycho-therapy (IPT), psychoeducation, support, physical exercise, and other treatments (e.g., music therapy), although the researchers noted that results should be interpreted with caution due to the small number of controlled studies of psychodynamic therapy and interpersonal psychotherapy.[13] Cognitive behavioral therapy has been the most widely studied stand-alone (i.e., without medication) treatment for depression, with studies of IPT in conjunction with medication producing equally positive results.

Generalized anxiety disorder (GAD) is the most common anxiety disorder diagnosis studied in controlled intervention trials of CBT. Overall, research has found CBT to be more effective than waitlist controls and TAU for GAD and other anxiety disorders (e.g., panic disorder, unspecified anxiety disorder, etc.).[13–15] Studies comparing CBT to other active treatments for anxiety are mixed. In a meta-analysis of 14 RCTs investigating the efficacy of CBT for GAD in older adults published between 1996 and 2015,[15] 5 of the intervention studies compared CBT to active controls, which included nondirective psy-chotherapy, discussion group, acceptance and commitment therapy (ACT), and escitalo-pram. In this study, CBT was slightly more effective than active controls at reducing excessive and uncontrollable worry at the end of treatment, though this finding was nonsignificant, and the outcomes were equivalent to other therapies at 6-month follow-up. Another meta-analysis of 12 studies, with all but 4 focused primarily on GAD, found a small significant difference in favor of CBT at 6-month follow-up but not at 3-month or 12-month follow-up.[13] Finally, a third meta-analysis of nine randomized control trials studying the effectiveness of CBT for any late-life anxiety disorder found that CBT was superior at reducing anxiety symptoms compared to active control conditions, which included supportive therapy, a discussion group, and weekly telephone calls.[15] Moreover, the studies included in this meta-analysis allowed for inclusion of patients with comorbid depression, and CBT outperformed the active control conditions in reducing depressive symptoms as well.

The literature on CBT for the treatment of psychotic, bipolar, and trauma-related disorders in older adults is scarce. Treatment for psychotic and bipolar disorders warrants pharmacotherapy and typically focuses on medication adherence, promoting daily routine and consistent sleep, basic coping skills training, and relapse prevention plans.[16–19] Similar to treatment of unipolar depression, standard components of CBT are applicable to bipolar depression in the adult population,[20] and the solid research support for CBT in the treatment of unipolar depression in older adults suggests that it may also be effective at treating bipolar depression in this population.[18] Most of the literature on treatment of trauma-related disorders in older adults describes clinical experiences, case studies, and small pilot studies[21] that have focused on prolonged exposure therapy (PE), a trauma-specific cognitive behavioral treatment. Prolonged exposure therapy includes psychoeducation, breathing retraining, imaginal exposure, and in vivo exposure.[22] The small amount of literature on PE in the treatment of trauma-related disorders among older adults is promising.[22,23]

Although not as extensively researched as depression and anxiety, CBT has been shown to be effective in treating insomnia. Behavioral components in CBT for insomnia (i.e., CBT-I) include a combination of sleep hygiene, stimulus control, sleep restriction, and relaxation training to improve sleep behaviors, and the cognitive component uses cognitive restructuring to challenge distorted thoughts that often contribute to poor perceived sleep quality. One systematic review and two meta-analyses of intervention studies investigating treatment for insomnia in older adults indicate that CBT-I is effective at improving sleep quality in this population.[24–26] The first meta-analysis included six RCTs of CBT-I in older adults and found that CBT-I had a small but positive effect on sleep, with the largest improvement occurring for sleep maintenance.[25] Another meta-analysis evidenced CBT-I to be significantly more efficacious than relaxation training but equivalent to behavioral treatment.[26] For further reading on using CBT for insomnia with older adults, readers are encouraged to review the article written by Bélanger, LeBlanc, and Morin, which provides a session-by-session description of implementation as well as important adaptations for this population.[27]

Cognitive behavioral therapy for Chronic Pain (CBT-CP) is now a standard treatment for chronic pain, but the research on CBT-CP for older adults lags compared to the research in working-aged adults.[28] Lunde, Nordhus, and Pallesen found only 12 studies published between 1975 and 2008 to include in their meta-analysis of research on cognitive and behavioral interventions for the treatment of chronic pain in older adults, and 5 of those studies did not have a control group.[29] They found that cognitive and behavioral interventions were effective at reducing self-reported pain, with a small significant effect on physical functioning but no effect on depression or medication use. A more recently published randomized controlled trial of CBT-CP in older adults found the treatment to be effective at reducing disability, pain distress, and unhelpful pain beliefs.[30]

Research investigating the effectiveness of CBT delivered in formats other than individual face-to-face therapy has shown promise. Group CBT has shown to be effective for the treatment of depression and anxiety in older adults.[31–35] Internet (iCBT),[36–39] telehealth,[40,41] and telephone-delivered CBT[42] have also resulted in positive effects in the treatment of anxiety, depression, insomnia, and pain in older adults, expanding services from a traditional outpatient clinic to the home. Researchers and clinicians have also successfully implemented CBT with older adults in long-term care,[43] in primary care,[44,45] and in individuals' homes.[46]

Patient Selection and Appropriate Patient Population

Cognitive behavioral therapy is appropriate for older adults presenting with symptoms of depression and anxiety, and can effectively decrease emotional distress in individuals with a range of medical conditions, including chronic obstructive pulmonary disease,[32,44,47] heart failure,[44,47–49] Parkinson's disease,[50,51] stroke,[52,53] and acute illnesses.[31] Underserved, rural-dwelling, physically frail, low-resource, African American older adults benefit from CBT as well, with research evidencing decreases in depression and anxiety as well as positive patient satisfaction with treatment.[46,54,55] With appropriate modifications, CBT can also be used to treat depression and anxiety in older adults with mild to moderate dementia.[56–61]

Treatment effectiveness may vary depending on a number of factors. Research suggests that CBT has smaller effects for patients with major depression compared to less severe mood disorders.[10] Similarly, regarding CBT for anxiety, Hundt and colleagues found that lower initial anxiety and worry predicted better outcomes,[62] though this contrasts with findings from earlier research.[63] Research on the effectiveness of CBT for treatment of anxiety in older versus working-aged adults is mixed. Specifically, Conti and colleagues found that adults aged 50–64 with anxiety may benefit less from CBT compared to those aged 65 and older, which they predicted may be due to added stressors associated with working and other factors. In contrast, Gould and colleagues suggest that CBT may be less effective at treating anxiety in older adults compared to working-aged adults,[13] which is supported by a meta-analysis of 22 randomized control trials that compared CBT for GAD in working-aged adults to older adults.[64] Kishita and Laidlaw conducted a qualitative content analysis of the treatment protocols used in the studies included in their meta-analysis of 22 studies and concluded that the protocols for older adults used standard CBT with a few procedural modifications (e.g., use of mnemonics, simplification of homework and terminology used in sessions) and did not utilize relevant gerontological theories (e.g., selective optimization with compensation) that could have enhanced treatment effectiveness.[64]

Although CBT can be effectively used in ethnically diverse populations, CBT for anxiety may be less effective for African Americans compared to Caucasians.[65] Older adults with lower educational attainment and those who use ineffective active coping strategies at baseline may show less improvement in depression compared to their counterparts.[66] Factors associated with greater improvements in depression include openness to new experiences, greater internal locus of control, lower negative impact of stressful life events, assignment of blame for stressful events on others, and use of emotional support from others.[66] Regarding cognitive functioning, any error in orientation on the Mini Mental State Examination has been shown to be associated with a lower response to CBT, and executive dysfunction that does not improve with treatment is associated with poorer outcomes.[67] Completion of homework[62,63,68] and use of memory aids (e.g., troubleshooting calls, homework reminders, weekly reviews) can improve treatment effectiveness.

Conducting CBT with Older Adults

In this section, an overview of 20-session CBT is presented. Readers are encouraged to use this as a guide, with flexibility in duration and length based on provider judgment. An optional 4–5 sessions can be added between standard modules when core belief work is indicated.

Table 4.1 Overview of CBT for Older Adults

Session 1 Initial Session
✓ Conduct clinical interview
✓ Risk assessment
✓ Self-report measures (e.g., PHQ-9)

Sessions 2–3 Orientation and Psychoeducation
✓ Orient to CBT
✓ Introduce ABC model and elicit examples from client
✓ Introduce basic CBT model
✓ Assign practice assignment (CBT model handout)
✓ Therapist works on expanded CBT model and case formulation in preparation for sessions 4–5

Sessions 4–5 Goal Setting
✓ Establish goals
✓ Provide case formulation to patient
✓ Provide expanded CBT model
✓ Present skills toolbox
✓ Describe outcome tracking

Sessions 6–9
✓ Psychoeducation on connection between activity and mood (e.g., downward and upward spirals)
✓ Activity monitoring
✓ Activity scheduling and review
✓ Problem-solving model
✓ Assign practice assignments

Sessions 10–15 Thinking Skills Module
✓ Reintroduce the ABC model
✓ Define negative automatic thoughts (NATs) and elicit examples from client
✓ Socratic dialogue in session to begin challenging thoughts
✓ Introduce Three-Column Dysfunctional Thought Record
✓ Psychoeducation on types of cognitive errors
✓ Introduce thought challenging techniques
✓ Introduce Five-Column Dysfunctional Thought Record
✓ Assign practice assignments

Table 4.1 (cont.)

Sessions 16–18 Feelings Skills
✓ Introduce tension diary and relaxation training
　　o Progressive Muscle Relaxation (PMR)
　　o Diaphragmatic breathing
　　o Guided imagery

✓ Assign practice assignments

Sessions 19–20 Termination and Relapse Prevention
✓ Reviews progress and goals
✓ Readminister outcome measures
✓ Create relapse prevention plan
✓ Process relationship

+ 4–5 Sessions Core Beliefs Modification (optional)
✓ Use techniques to identify core beliefs
　　o Downward arrow
　　o Developmental approach

✓ Introduce techniques to challenge core beliefs
　　o Positive data log
　　o As If
　　o Continuum technique

Session 1: Initial Intake Session

An initial clinical interview provides the first step in understanding the client from a biopsychosocial perspective. The therapist begins by focusing on the present by asking the client about the frequency, severity, and duration of current problem(s), which serves a dual purpose of informing a diagnostic impression and providing a baseline assessment of symptoms. The therapist may choose to administer self-report measures to supplement the clinical interview to be collected at the beginning or end of the session, or measures can be incorporated into the interview itself with the therapist verbally asking the screening questions (e.g., Patient Health Questionnaire-9 [PHQ-9][69]; Geriatric Depression Scale-15 [GDS-15][70]; Geriatric Anxiety Inventory [GAI][71]). If self-report measures are not completed at the initial intake, it is recommended they be administered at the beginning of the next session, as they will serve as a measure of treatment outcome. Self-report measures of NATs, such as the Cognitive Distortions Scale (CDS), can be administered to begin identifying problematic cognitions,[72] although this measure has yet to be validated in older adult samples.

Another focus of the intake is on understanding the context in which the problem(s) is (are) occurring, such as current stressors, general coping style/pattern (problem-focused, avoidant, etc.), quality and quantity of social support, and religious/spiritual beliefs. A risk assessment, including risk of suicide, homicide, and elder abuse or neglect, is conducted. The therapist also gathers information about the client's past mental health history (i.e., diagnosis and treatment) and psychosocial history, particularly asking about life events that may have shaped longstanding core beliefs. It is also prudent to note sensory impairments or other medical or physical conditions that may require adaptation. When working with older adults, it is important to attend to how unique age-related factors may intersect with elements of the CBT model. These factors include changes in health, role investments, cohort beliefs, intergenerational linkages, and the sociocultural context.[73]

Based on initial intake with Mr. John Doe, the following synthesis was developed:

Case Example – John Doe

Current

Mr. Doe is a 70-year-old, widowed White man who was referred by his psychiatric provider for individual psychotherapy at an outpatient mental health clinic for major depressive disorder (MDD), recurrent, severe. Depressive symptoms are notable for almost daily low mood, anhedonia, lack of motivation, poor appetite, fluctuating sleeping (sleeping too much or too little), and intermittent suicidal ideation (SI) (sometimes with plan, but no intent). His PHQ-9 score was 16, indicating moderately severe depressive symptoms. In addition, he presents with a remote history of alcohol use disorder and current nicotine use disorder. He is under the care of a psychiatric provider and currently prescribed bupropion, sertraline, and mirtazapine. Past mental health treatment includes remote inpatient admission for alcohol use with sobriety of 30 years. He worked with a prior therapist on several occasions over the last 10 years, focused on coping with current stressors. Therapy ended due to the therapist's retirement.

Mr. Doe made one suicide attempt in his 30s by overdose of medications while intoxicated. He was last psychiatrically hospitalized one year prior to this intake for severe depression without suicidal ideation. Historically, he has reported intermittent SI, ranging from death ideation ("I would be better off dead"; "There's no point in living") to SI with plan, throughout different periods of his life. He denied SI at initial intake. Current reasons for living include his son, grandchildren, and a promise he made to his deceased wife. At the time of intake, he was deemed to be at low acute risk but with several chronic risk factors. Ongoing monitoring of SI, plan, and intent, and reasons for living would occur throughout treatment, including development of a safety plan.[74]

Several psychosocial stressors and life events are notable. Mr. Doe lost his wife of many decades to cancer within the last two years. He lives in subsidized housing and has chronic financial strain. He has some conflict with adult biological and stepchildren, although he noted good relationships with some of his children. He is largely socially isolated, though he talks with neighbors in his apartment complex. With respect to functioning, he currently drives, is independent for all activities of daily living, and ambulates independently. Due to financial limitations, he does not have money for leisure activities associated with a cost (e.g., movies, taking public transportation). Major health contributions include severe chronic obstructive pulmonary disease (COPD). Mr. Doe was raised as a Catholic and believes in a God but is currently "not religious."

Relevant History

Mr. Doe was born to and raised in a working class family in a suburb close to a major city in the United States. His parents were married, and he had one older sister, with whom he remains in touch. He described his childhood as "difficult" with frequent emotional abuse by a father who was often intoxicated. He described his mother as "a saint," and she provided caring and warmth to Mr. Doe and his sister. Mr. Doe enlisted in the military while in high school to escape his family environment. He served for five years during the Vietnam era working in aircraft maintenance and did not see combat. He spoke of his military experience favorably and appreciated that it afforded him a way to complete his general education diploma (GED). Mr. Doe was honorably discharged and returned to the states where he worked in occupations involving manual labor. He was married to his first wife for 10 years and had five children. They were divorced amicably. He met his second wife while recovering from alcohol abuse at a residential facility where she worked as a healthcare provider. They did not have children together, but he helped raise two stepdaughters with his wife. He described their marriage as a "wonderful partnership."

Sessions 2–3: Orientation and Psychoeducation

Session 2: Orientation. The initial session establishes a solid foundation by orienting the client to treatment. The therapist elicits the client's expectations for therapy, followed by providing information about the current therapy. Core aspects of CBT that are discussed with the client include the *what* and *how* of therapy. The *what* of therapy includes a focus on the present (although core beliefs informed by past events are incorporated) and intervention at the level of thoughts, behaviors, and emotions. The *how* includes orienting the client to the therapy's collaborative and time-limited nature, goal setting, use of outcome tracking, and need for practice outside of session.

    Introducing the CBT Model. The basic CBT model describes the connection between an event, thoughts, emotions, behaviors, and physiological response. First, the therapist describes the cognitive-behavioral model, noting the bi-directionality of the basic CBT model, and uses a general example to illustrate it (e.g., describe an event [running late] with corresponding thought ["I mess up everything"], emotion [anger, sadness, self-hate], behavior [stay in the house for the rest of the day], and physiological response, if present) (Figure 4.1). After presenting a general example, the therapist presents an example that is reflective of the client's presenting problem, providing additional examples as needed.

    Mr. Doe voiced the belief "I will never feel better." Using the basic CBT model, Mr. Doe and the therapist identified the event (loss of wife) → thought ("I will never feel better") →emotion (sadness, hopelessness) + behavior (does not leave apartment) + physiological response (slowed down sensation). By the end of the second session, the therapist and client collaboratively complete a blank CBT model worksheet based on a recent life event. The therapist should assess the client's understanding of the elements of the model and their connections. At the end of the session, the therapist assigns the first homework assignment, which is to review the basic cognitive behavioral model (Appendix A).

    Session 3: The expanded cognitive behavioral model is presented to the client once the basic model is understood. The expanded model incorporates early life experiences, the development of schemas, and the role of core beliefs. This information often serves to help answer questions related to the nature and function of patterns of behavior over time and the tendency for clients to become stuck in unhelpful patterns of responding to internal and

A Situation	B Beliefs	C Emotion, Behavior, Physiological response

Figure 4.1 Basic CBT Model ("ABC" Model)

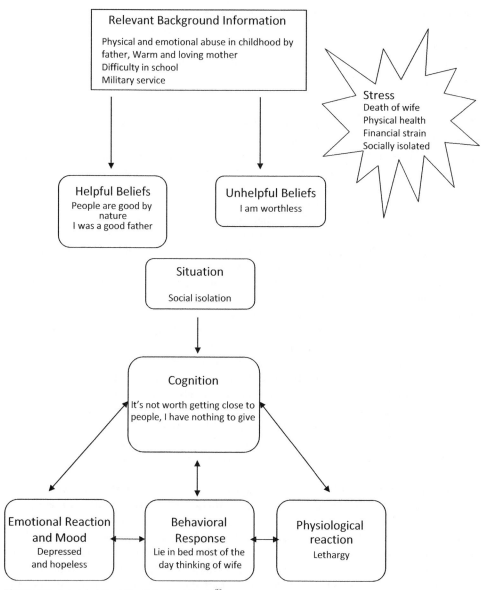

Figure 4.2 Expanded Cognitive Behavioral Model[76]

external stressors. The therapist's role is to guide the client through the model, elicit understanding, and present relevant examples based on the client's life.

Figure 4.2 illustrates the expanded model for Mr. Doe. Mr. Doe's negative early life experiences shaped the development of negative schemas about himself, others, and the world, known as the negative cognitive triad.[75] Mr. Doe believed that he was worthless and carried minimal intrinsic value as a human. He was hypersensitive to evidence that the people in his life no longer cared for him. He often self-isolated, reducing opportunities for connectedness and belonging. When his wife of many years died, Mr. Doe's life fell apart. His longstanding depression became severe and refractory to medication, and he was hospitalized for self-neglect and passive suicidal ideation. At initial intake, he voiced a desire to "feel better" and "think differently" but did not possess the skills to foster changes in thinking and behavior.

Sessions 4–5: Goal Setting, Skill Toolbox, and Case Formulation

Session 4: Goal Setting is important because it provides a measurable index of treatment success, and it also helps the client and therapist adhere to an agenda. Choosing 2–3 goals is ideal, as identifying too many goals can become overwhelming. Goals should be discrete, measurable, and concrete. Clients may generate vague goals at first, such as "I want to be happy" or "I want to not be depressed." Using the CBT framework, the therapist helps the client operationalize vague goals so that they can be tracked over the course of therapy (e.g., "I want to be happy" ➔ "I want to experience more positive emotions on more days"). Mr. Doe developed the following goals: "To engage in one meaningful activity per day" and "To learn how to talk back to my negative thoughts."

Outcome Tracking. Outcome tracking is a core feature of CBT. The easiest method for tracking symptoms includes collecting self-report measures of relevant symptoms at the beginning of therapy, throughout the therapy (~ 2–3 weeks), and at the conclusion of therapy. This provides a criterion for change demonstrating reduction of the frequency and intensity of symptoms. Graphing clients' change in outcomes over time can foster a sense of agency and direction. The client's subjective report, of course, is also a critical component of outcomes. Does the client believe the goals are being met? Because depression can bias self-report, it's important to also observe whether measurable improvement in goals matches the client's report. Therapist observations (e.g., greater awareness skills, flexibility in thinking), clients' application of skills in and out of sessions, and completion of homework assignments can be tracked. When working with older adults with cognitive impairment, proxy report of symptoms and functioning can also be used.[77]

Session 5: Case Formulation. The therapist's case formulation of the client begins at intake and serves as a living document, guiding therapy across the duration of treatment (Table 4.2). Case formulation aids the therapist in making sense of information hypothesized to be connected to the presenting problem(s). Cognitive behavioral therapy adopts a biopsychosocial framework, including biological (e.g., genetics, family history), social (e.g., learning history, family environment, important developmental experiences), and psychological factors (e.g., personality, resiliency). The client's helpful and unhelpful thinking (core beliefs), rules and assumptions (intermediary beliefs, conditional beliefs), and any compensatory strategies are identified and summarized. Acute and chronic stressors, which may be age-related in nature, are considered. At the end of the formulation, the therapist identifies several ABC sequences playing out in the client's daily life.

Below is a completed case formulation for Mr. Doe.

Skills Tool Box. The skills toolbox refers to the set of skills in CBT that comprise the active ingredients for change. They can be broken down into behavior, thinking, and feeling modules. The behavior module includes behavioral activation and problem-solving. The thinking module includes identifying NATs, challenging NATs, and challenging

Table 4.2 CBT Case Formulation[78]

Vulnerability Factors

Environmental
Physical and emotion abuse by father

Biological
Family history of depression and alcohol use disorder (father's side)

Psychological
Received little praise growing up; limited emotion regulation skills

Cultural
Mental health stigma in family

Beliefs

Helpful Beliefs
I try to be a good person, do no harm to anybody.

Unhelpful Beliefs
I am worthless; I am to blame for everything bad; I do not belong (in the world); I have little to offer others; I do not deserve happiness.

Unhelpful Rules and Assumptions
If I express my needs and emotions to others, I will be rejected.

Unhelpful Compensatory Strategies
Do not leave house for days; skip meals; decline social events; oversleep.

Stressors

Chronic Stressors
Live alone; chronic health conditions (COPD); financial strain.

Acute Stressors
Death of wife; recent disappointments by adult children and stepchildren

Situational Manifestations				
Situation	**NAT**	**Emotional Reaction**	**Physiological Reaction**	**Behavioral Activation**
My daughter did not call me	*"She doesn't care about me."*	*Depressed, hopeless, unlovable*	*Feel slowed down*	*Lie in bed all day, "talk" to deceased wife. Do not make myself dinner.*
Wife's death	*"I have nothing left to live for."*	*Depressed, hopeless*	*Slowed down*	*Ruminate about loss; stay at home; stop volunteering at cat shelter.*

dysfunctional core beliefs. The feeling tools module includes gaining awareness of tension and tension triggers, and learning relaxation skills.

Where to Begin. The therapist uses clinical judgment, based on the case formulation, to select the most appropriate module to begin with in therapy. When working with clients who have more severe depression, it is best to start with behavioral skills first, as clients tend to have a more immediate mood lifting effect and increased motivation. Mildly depressed patients or those who have adjustment disorders have been noted in the treatment literature to respond well to thinking skills first.[1] Choice of the initial intervention may be influenced by the client's treatment goals. For example, if a client's primary goal is to slow down thinking and reduce anxiety, then starting with the feeling skills to lower arousal level may be clinically indicated. In the case of Mr. Doe, the therapist elected to start with behavioral skills, due to moderately severe depression, with the hope that behavioral activation would provide a modest decline in depressive symptoms and enhance motivation for the thinking skills module. For the purpose of this chapter, the reader will be guided through a course of CBT beginning with the behavioral skills module.

Structure and Flow. Cognitive behavioral therapy sessions are structured but versatile, meaning that the therapist should adjust and adapt to the client based on the therapy goals (whether immediate or longer term). For example, a client may enter session acutely distressed due to a recent life stressor. In this case, the therapist should respond to the immediate distress, while still practicing within the CBT framework (assessing thoughts, emotions, and behaviors in the context of the stressor, adding a relaxation exercise to the beginning of the session, etc.). The general structure of the sessions is as follows: (1) Check-in with symptoms and problems from the interim between sessions; (2) Review the practice assignment from the previous week; (3) Set the day's agenda by identifying which problem area/goal to focus on; (4) Apply the cognitive model to elicit the client's thoughts, emotions, and behaviors in the context of the current problem or situation; (5) Provide new content or existing material as needed to foster problem-solving, recognize negative thinking and challenge it, and/or effect behavior change based on the problem at hand; and (6) Assign new homework in line with the client's immediate or longer-term goals.

Sessions 6–9: Behavior Skills Module

Session 6: Behavioral Activation. Behavior therapy comprises a set of behavioral interventions with the goal of demonstrating the connection between activity level and mood, decreasing avoidance behaviors, and fostering problem-solving skills. In Session 6, when initiating BT, the therapist provides psychoeducation on the connection between activity and mood through presentation of the downward spiral. The downward spiral describes how a stressor triggers depressed mood, which results in activity reduction and fewer opportunities for pleasant events. This initial withdrawal results in a worsening of mood, which, in turn, leads to more withdrawal from activities in daily life, which results in a chronically depressed state. Clients often easily relate to this cycle.

Next, the therapist explains that part of therapy will involve reversing the downward spiral by increasing activity levels (Figure 4.3). Two types of events are highlighted: pleasant events and masterful events. Pleasant events provide response-contingent positive reinforcement and improve mood and motivation. Masterful events produce a sense of accomplishment and purpose, and increase feelings of hopefulness and agency. For the first assignment, the client is asked to complete the Activity Monitoring Form. **Activity monitoring** is a process by which the client is asked to track day-to-day activity and its related sense of pleasure (P), mastery (M), and mood.[1-10] The client's monitoring provides a baseline measure of activity and mood levels, as well as patterns of activity (e.g., particularly low activity levels during certain times of the day) and their connection to mood. Below is an example of Mr. Doe's initial activity monitoring form.

Table 4.3 Activity Monitoring Log

Monday	Tuesday	Wednesday	Thursday	Friday	Saturday	Sunday
Read book P (5); M (1); Mood (2)	Went to grocery store P (2); M (5); Mood (4)				Went to my sister's house. P (7); M (6); Mood (7)	Talked to neigh-bor P (4); M (2); Mood (5)

Pleasure (P) 1–10 (1= little pleasure, 10 = much pleasure; Mastery 1–10 (1 = little mastery, 10 = high mastery); Mood 1–10 (1 = very depressed; 10 = very happy; 5 = neutral)

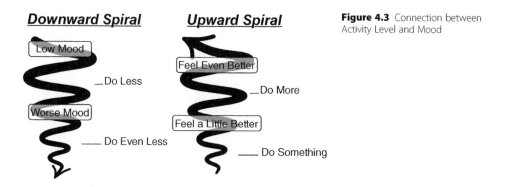

Figure 4.3 Connection between Activity Level and Mood

Session 7: At the next session, the therapist and client review the Activity Monitoring Form, which is used to assist with generating a list of pleasant and masterful events. The therapist queries the client regarding patterns noticed, such as times of day with relatively lower or higher activity levels, and whether the client derived pleasure or a sense of accomplishment from the activities. The therapist highlights the connection between activity levels and mood. When considering Mr. Doe's completed activity monitoring form, the therapist noticed several patterns. First, Mr. Doe engaged in few activities. This is not uncommon when first beginning behavioral activation and is consistent with the behavioral model of depression. Limited activity engagement should be noted and tied back to the downward spiral, as a way to provide education and reinforcement of the link between mood and behavior. Second, Mr. Doe's log features three days on which he either did not complete the log or did not engage in any activities. In these instances, when part of the log is blank, the therapist queries the client to determine the cause. In cases of nonadherence, the therapist should assess barriers and facilitators to homework completion and problem-solve accordingly.

In discussion with Mr. Doe, the therapist learned that he did not engage in any activities on those three days. This had become a pattern for Mr. Doe in which he would build momentum for a few days and then lose momentum. Several approaches were used to address these gaps, including assessing what was occurring during these time periods (e.g., heavy periods of rumination where he would feel "stuck" on the couch), implementing activity scheduling (see below), and eventually applying thought challenging to foster more flexibility to respond to overwhelming grief, rumination, and hopelessness. Finally, the therapist noted activities the client reported deriving pleasure or mastery from (e.g., "Went to sister's house"), as this information would inform the next skill – activity scheduling.

Activity Scheduling is a process by which activities are scheduled into the client's week. The principle behind this approach is that increased activity will result in improved mood and activation. The therapist and client identify a list of pleasant and masterful events to add to daily life. Addressing barriers (e.g., logistical barriers, such as time of day, access to transportation, availability of hobbies and activities in the environment) ahead of time is helpful. It is typical for clients to express "not feeling" like engaging in activities, in which case the therapist reminds the client that part of reversing the downward spiral is focusing on action, even if the action is contrary to mood. The therapist and client work collaboratively to schedule the identified activities into the Activity Scheduling Form for the next week. Use of a standardized pleasant events list such as the Pleasant Event Schedule[79] or the California Older Person's Pleasant Event Schedule[80] is helpful when clients have difficulty generating a list of pleasant events. Another helpful tool is Karlin's 4-A Approach to Activity Scheduling: (1) Assess types of activities the client did in the past, (2) Assess level of functioning related to engaging in activities, (3) Assess actual versus perceived level of physical activity, and (4) Adapt activities to current level of functioning. Many clients need help with breaking down activity engagement.[3]

Next, therapist and client create an activity-scheduling log (Table 4.4). Clients will denote which days they engage in a particular event and provide an end-of-day mood rating. Below is an example of Mr. Doe's activity-scheduling form.

Sessions 8–9: The therapist and client will continue with activity scheduling for Sessions 8–9, monitoring activity level and troubleshooting barriers. Problem-solving (discussed below) is also introduced and implemented.

Problem-Solving Skills. Problem-solving can be introduced at any point during the behavioral skills module, as judged appropriate by the therapist. Clients will arrive to therapy with varying levels of problem-solving abilities. Some clients may have deficient problem-solving skills, and for them problem-solving skill building will be necessary and is typically introduced early. Others may have good problem-solving skills, but heightened stress and distorted cognitions may impede problem-solving abilities. Problem-solving skills involve multiple steps beginning with (1) Identification of the problem; (2) Outlining goals; (3) Listing possible solutions and pros and cons for each; (4) Selecting a solution; and (5) Evaluating the consequences.[81] Problem-solving skills are commonly applied throughout CBT. Basic problem-solving skills are often needed in conjunction with activity scheduling to troubleshoot barriers and break down steps. To address unhelpful thinking patterns, problem-solving skills may be applied for managing stressors in the moment and planning to cope effectively ahead of time in anticipation of challenging situations.[82] Problem-solving has the added benefit of challenging rigid thinking, by having the client engage in more flexible thinking about their daily stressors and possible solutions. See Appendix B for a sample problem-solving worksheet.

Sessions 10–15: Thinking Skills Module

Session 10: Recognition and Awareness Building. The Thinking Skills Module is rooted in cognitive therapy. The first step of this module is to help the client gain awareness and recognition of unhelpful thinking patterns, which is accomplished with a combination of psychoeducation, Socratic dialogue, and completion of practice assignments. The clinician begins Session 10 by re-introducing the role of thoughts in precipitating and perpetuating distress, through review of the ABC model, and by eliciting current examples from the

Table 4.4 Activity Scheduling Form

Pleasant or Masterful Events

	Monday	Tuesday	Wednesday	Thursday	Friday	Saturday	Sunday
Go for walk				X		X	
Go to coffee shop	X						
Empty and organize three boxes in closet		X	X				
Go to senior center							
Watch a movie				X			
Do dishes playing music					X		
Listen to audiobook						X	
Go to church							X
Mood 1–10 (1 = very depressed; 10 = very happy; 5 = neutral)							

49

client's daily life. Then, the therapist and client work together to identify NATs. It is helpful to redefine NATs for the client and provide examples, such as "I can't handle it," "I fail at everything," "Things are out of control," "I'll never be able to get this done," "Something bad is sure to happen," "I always mess up." Negative automatic thoughts are readily identified through the presence of cognitive errors (Table 4.6).

The therapist reviews the ABC model and asks the client to identify a recent event or stressor. For example, Ms. Jones' identified stressor is finding it increasingly difficult to leave her house due to fear of falling. This fear developed after she fell in a grocery store approximately two months earlier. She identified the beliefs, "I will fall and injure myself" and "I can't do it." Her emotional response was anxiety and dread, and her physiological response was the sensation of having a knot in her stomach. She reported that the behavioral consequence was to stay in the home and decline social invitations. When examining Ms. Jones' thoughts, catastrophizing and absolutist language were identified as cognitive errors (Table 4.6). Returning to Mr. Doe, his NATs included "I am worthless," "I am unlovable," and "I don't deserve to feel better." These cognitive errors are classified as emotional reasoning, labeling, and overgeneralization.

After reviewing the ABC model, the Three-Column Dysfunctional Thought Record, which helps clients identify NATs, is introduced. In Column A, the client lists the antecedent, usually a situation, stressor, or event. Next, in Column B, the client lists "What I tell myself" or the client's interpretation of the situation, followed by the emotional response (Column C). If clients have difficulty identifying their thoughts, the therapist can have the patient identify the stressor (A) followed by the emotional response (C), and then work backwards to the thought (B). The client rates the strength of their NATs from 0 (not strong at all) to 100 (strongest possible) and emotional response from 0 (not strong at all) to 100 (strongest possible).

At the end of Session 10, clients are instructed to take home the Three-Column Dysfunctional Thought Record and complete one row a day for the next week.

Session 11: Types of Negative Automatic Thoughts. Beginning in Session 11, different types of cognitive errors are introduced that describe unhelpful patterns of thinking exemplified in the client's NATs (Table 4.6). Clinical researchers have defined common cognitive errors characteristic across diagnostic categories.[83,84] Therapists are familiar with these errors and, through psychoeducation and Socratic dialogue, help the client to recognize, label, and challenge cognitive errors. Table 4.6 provides definitions of each type of cognitive error and example excerpts based on the case study of Mr. Doe

Table 4.5 Three-Column Dysfunctional Thought Record

Date	Situation (A)	Belief (B)	Emotion (C)
	What happened?	What did you tell yourself? (Rate on a 0–100 scale)	What emotion(s) did you experience? (Rate on a 0–100 scale)
Mr. John Doe	I didn't leave my house today	I am a failure	Hopelessness (100%); sadness (100%); anxiety (80%).

Table 4.6 List of Cognitive Errors[84,85]

Belief	Label for Client	Description	Examples
Arbitrary Inference	Jumping to Conclusions	Drawing a specific conclusion in the absence of evidence.	
	Two Types: A. Mind Reading	A. Mind reading – drawing conclusions without evidence that someone is responding negatively to you.	A. Adult son does not call this week; assume, "They don't care about me." Coworker passing in the hallway does not say hello; tell self, "They must not like me," "Did I do something wrong?"
	B. Fortune-Telling	B. Predicting a future event will turn out negatively without evidence or minimal evidence.	B. When thinking about going to a social event, think "I can't do anything right. I will mess this up too." "I never do well socially. Everyone will be able to tell, and I will look like a fool."
Selective Abstraction	Mental Filter	Focusing on a detail out of its context while ignoring more salient information. Individuals will focus on negative or threatening aspects of reality and ignore or discount positive aspects.	When out at a social situation, only focus on part of the night that didn't go as planned; say to self, "The night was a complete failure."
Dichotomous Reasoning	Black-and-White Thinking	Propensity to categorize all experiences in one of two categories.	"Unless I do something perfectly, it is not good enough; if I can't do things completely independently, I would rather not do them."
Overgeneralization	Overinterpreting	Drawing a conclusion in the absence of substantiating evidence.	Giving up on an activity because you struggled with it ("I am never doing this again"); running late for an appointment, you think, "I always mess things up. I can't do anything right."

Table 4.6 (cont.)

Belief	Label for Client	Description	Examples
Personalization	Personalization	Propensity to relate external events to oneself.	Adult daughter is suffering from drug addiction; client tells himself, "It's my fault she turned out this way."
Catastrophizing	Catastrophizing	A propensity to think about the worst possible outcomes for situations.	"I failed at this thing; I will fail at all things."
Magnification and Minimization	Making a Mountain Out of a Molehill (Magnification) Tuning Out the Positive (Minimization)	Either exaggerating or downplaying the personal significance of an event.	"I forgot something from the store; I must have dementia."
Negative Imperatives	"Tyranny of the Shoulds"	A precise and fixed idea of how things ought to be in the world ("should" and "must" statements).	"I must clean the house to a certain standard"; "I should feel better by now."
Emotional Reasoning	Emotional Reasoning	Using feels as a basis for the facts of a situation.	"I feel hopeless, so the situation is hopeless."
Labeling	Namecalling	Attaching a negative label to yourself or others.	"I am a bad partner"; "I am a failure."

and other exemplar cases. A copy may be provided to the client to aid in identifying cognitive errors.

Sessions 11–12: Challenging NATs. In Session 11 or 12, the therapist engages in Socratic dialogue aimed at clarifying, exploring, and challenging thinking patterns, and introduces skills to challenge NATs. Socratic dialogue refers to statements and questions that are collaborative, inquisitive, empirical, and guided, and are used by the therapist to enhance flexibility in thinking and facilitate discovery and insight on behalf of the client (Table 4.7). Once the client has gained greater awareness of thinking patterns, the therapist describes strategies to challenge dysfunctional thoughts, usually in Session 12.

Strategies to Challenge Dysfunctional Thoughts

Examining the evidence is a simple way of challenging cognitive errors. This technique asks the client to examine the evidence confirming and disconfirming the belief in question. Describing evidence as facts that can be held up in a court of law can help differentiate emotional reasoning (which often feels very real) from fact-based reasoning. For example, if

Table 4.7 Socratic Question Bank[82,91]

Eliciting Thoughts
What goes through your head when a problem begins?
What's going through your mind right now?
What do you say to yourself when this occurs?
What did you say to yourself?
What comes to mind when you think about that event?

Linking Thoughts to Emotions and Behavior
What is it like to have this belief?
When you have the thought X, how do you feel?
When you have the thought X, what do you do?

Enlist Collaboration
Does this fit your experience?
How does this sound to you? Tell me if this sounds correct?

Challenging Thoughts
What is the evidence for and against this belief?
What is another way of looking at the situation?
What is the effect of holding this belief?
How does it help you to think this way? What would a trusted friend or family member say?
What might you tell a trusted friend or family member when this thought occurs?
What aspects might you be overlooking or leaving out?
How does maintaining this thought serve you?
What could you do differently to manage those emotions?
What else might be involved here?
What is the evidence to support your view?
So if what you're saying is true, then X always happens?
So if what you're saying is true, you are entirely (useless, worthless, unlovable)? Is there any evidence suggesting otherwise? Are there any situations when you feel useful, lovable, or worthwhile?
Have you considered other possible causes?
What makes this situation a problem?
Have you ever felt like this before and responded in a helpful way? What happened that time?
How would this strategy play out over a longer period of time?

a client concludes, "I mess everything up," the client will be asked to evaluate the facts supporting and disputing this belief. Often, the belief is neutralized quickly using this approach because the facts supporting the belief are minimal, and the belief stems from one or more cognitive errors used when interpreting the situation.

The following exchange is an example of Socratic dialogue with Mr. Doe, which uses the technique of examining the evidence:

MR. DOE: My life is worthless.

THERAPIST: That's a very powerful statement that relates to a lot of your current suffering. I would like to try something new today. I would like to begin working together to challenge that thought. Would you be willing to try that today?

MR. DOE: Yeah, sure.

THERAPIST: First, I want us to look at the thought and test it factually. When I say "fact," what I mean is something that could be held up in a court of law. Many of our beliefs or thoughts are based on feelings or emotions but not on facts. The emotions and feelings are important, but for this exercise, I want to focus on the facts behind your thoughts. Does that make sense? We're going to focus on the factual evidence for and against your thought.

MR. DOE: Yes, I think I understand.

THERAPIST: Mr. Doe, when you consider the thought, "I am worthless," what evidence to you have for and against this thought?

MR. DOE: I have nothing to live for. That's why I am worthless.

THERAPIST: What I am hearing is that when you consider the thought, "I am worthless," another thought comes up, which is, "I have nothing to live for." These are both very important thoughts to consider. It's meaningful that they come up together, too. Let's go back to the first thought. What fact supports the belief, "I am worthless"?

MR. DOE: I am alone.

THERAPIST: Can you be more specific? What do you mean by being alone?

MR. DOE: My wife. She's gone.

THERAPIST: Your wife's passing has impacted you greatly. This is a palpable and painful reality for you. You are telling me that because you are alone, you are worthless? Is that correct?

MR. DOE: Yes, because I am alone, I am worthless.

THERAPIST: Are you completely alone? Is there anyone in your life?

MR. DOE: Well, there are some. My sister and my two sons. They call me.

THERAPIST: What does it mean to you that your sister and sons call you? Does that affect your feelings of worth?

MR. DOE: I know they care, but I still feel worthless.

THERAPIST: You said earlier that you feel worthless because you are alone, but what you mean more specifically is that you feel worthless because you lost the person who gave you a sense of purpose. You also note here that you have people in your life currently who care about you. Is that correct?

MR. DOE: Yes, I have some people.

THERAPIST: Is there any evidence against the belief, "I am worthless?"

MR. DOE: I try to do good in the world. I try to not do harm. I was a good father. I am not completely alone.

THERAPIST: How do these things inform the belief of "I am worthless?"

MR. DOE: Well, I guess I am not completely worthless. I have some good qualities. I am not completely alone, but I miss my wife.

Examine the Language Used. In mental health conditions, self-talk often becomes exaggerated and extreme in nature. The clinician helps the client recognize when extreme language is being used and question whether the extreme language is reflective of the situation at hand or an exaggeration. Extreme language can be identified when absolutist words are present, such as "always," "should," "everyone," "anything," "nothing," "everything," and "completely."

CLIENT (MR. DOE): I can't do anything right.

THERAPIST: I am noticing your use of extreme language here. You used the word "anything." We have been working on identifying when extreme language is used. Can you be more specific? What does this belief refer to specifically? Is it true you can't do anything right?

CLIENT (MR. DOE): I am angry that I forgot my homework. It just feels like I'm always messing up.

THERAPIST: Let's look at this situation in greater detail.

Here the therapist will challenge the absolutist terms of the statement by bringing in what the client does successfully. The therapist may also choose to utilize a second technique of considering the context in which this error occurred (e.g., client distracted by phone call, left homework on table, etc.) and use consideration of context to foster flexibility in thinking and a more realistic appraisal of the situation.

Examining the Consequence of Maintaining the Belief. The therapist will ask the client: "What is the consequence of holding this belief," or, stated a different way, "How does this thought serve you in the long run?" For example, Mr. Doe has the thought, "I'm too old to learn new ways of thinking." The therapist challenges this thought by examining the consequence of maintaining this belief, including the possibility that this thought may lead him to not engage in therapy, not complete practice assignments, or drop out of therapy. Many clients recognize that their unhelpful thoughts (NATs) serve to prolong distress. Acknowledging this reality can enhance motivation and willingness to modify thinking.

Consider Alternatives. This technique is used to gain flexibility in thinking from polarized, dichotomous thinking, to shades of gray and consideration of in-betweens. The therapist will ask clients to brainstorm as many alternative thoughts as possible, even if they do not buy into them yet. The point of the exercise is to generate different appraisals of realty that might challenge rigidly held black-and-white thinking. For example, Mrs. White is convinced that her friends at church are judging her and no longer like her. She began thinking this way when one of the women in her social circle did not ask her opinion on an upcoming church event and did not ask her to bring a dessert (which she normally is asked to do). Since this event, Mrs. White has avoided her social group in the hallway, has not picked up their phone calls, and has even missed a church meeting. As her therapist, you ask her to go back and describe the original situation and then describe alternative appraisals. She generates the following: "Perhaps the woman had a lot on her mind and forgot to ask me"; "Maybe she knew I was overwhelmed caregiving for my husband and wanted to give me a break"; "Maybe I offended her so she did not ask my opinion or to bring a dessert"; "It's possible I looked distracted at the time, so perhaps she thought I was not interested." Through Socratic dialogue, the therapist helps the client weigh the facts of each interpretation. Additionally, this is an example where problem-solving might be used to facilitate interpersonal skills to help Mrs. White mend the perceived rift between herself and her social circle.

Am I Including all the Information? When distressed, clients often view situations using tunnel vision with a hyper-focus on personal failure, magnifying the negative, and discrediting refuting information. For example, Mrs. White, from the example above, left out some important information when forming her original belief ("They don't like me"). Specifically, since that time, she has received several calls from her friends, yet this information was not assimilated into her interpretation of the event. She also did not consider the context (where did the event take place? was the room noisy? were there features of the setting that could explain her friend's response?). What about the woman in question – is there evidence to suggest this was a benign mistake on her part? Mrs. White also made a statement suggesting that she may have been distracted at the time of the conversation; how might this information be used to inform a more balanced appraisal of the situation? When challenging thoughts in this way, the therapist takes a genuinely inquisitive stance to help guide the client in increasing flexibility in thinking through dialogue.

Credit the positive is a simple technique that can meaningfully shift mood. Because depression entails a negative bias toward negative stimuli, helping clients credit the positive can foster more balanced thinking. Clients are asked to list 2–3 positive aspects of their daily life at the end of each day, which aids in attending to positive information. Clients may also be asked to consider positives, even when describing stressful situations or personal disappointments, by focusing on resiliency and surviving in spite of challenges.

Perspective taking is a simple, yet effective, cognitive strategy used to disrupt negative or anxious filters. The client is asked to consider how he or she would advise, respond, or react to a friend or family member in a similar position to the one being examined. For example, the client may be asked, "If your friend came to you with this particular situation, what would you tell him or her?" The goal of perspective taking is to draw awareness to how individuals often judge themselves more harshly and critically than others. The practice allows space for errors and mistakes, without attaching a stable, global, internal meaning to the self.

Acceptance, Self-Compassion, Forgiveness, and Gratitude. The practice of acceptance, self-compassion, forgiveness, and gratitude can be effective, particularly during negative life events when response-focused emotion regulation strategies are warranted.[86] These concepts have research support in their own right as independent intervention strategies and can be readily incorporated into CBT.[86–88] "Acceptance" refers to letting oneself experience unwanted internal experiences (e.g., thoughts or emotions) without judgment. Acceptance can be fostered by the clinician by encouraging the client to be present with the negative emotion(s), thought(s), or other unwanted physical sensations (e.g., panic symptoms) without adding judgment or interpretation to the experience. For example, Mr. Doe, who experienced significant grief, was encouraged to be present-focused and experience unwanted feelings of grief and loss in sessions without elaborating or expanding upon them. This practice allowed him to process the normative emotions of grief.

Self-compassion and gratitude lie within a similar vein to crediting the positive. The aim is to foster shifts in thinking from the largely negative to a more forgiving and thankful stance that is genuine and meaningful to the client. The practice of self-compassion and gratitude can be very helpful in situations in which the client has little control. At the heart of self-compassion is treating oneself kindly, like one would a friend or family member and decreasing over-identifying with perceived failures and losses.[89] The therapist may ask questions such as, "What would you tell a friend in your position?" Gratitude is often a foreign concept to clients, particularly among individuals with depression who experience a great deal of suffering in their lives. However, the powerful component of gratitude is that it can shift the individual from a wholly negative view to recognition of positive aspects in their lives. This is essential to changing the negative self-talk dominant in depressed states. Using a very simple exercise of listing 2–5 things that they feel grateful for at the end of the day can be an effective strategy to shift clients' negative filter. Finally, self- and other-forgiveness can be used when clients find themselves stuck in the past, regretting past mistakes or holding on to others' mistakes. Like gratitude, forgiveness can be harnessed through the active practice of being kind to oneself and others.

Behavioral experiments refer to planned experiential activities designed to test the validity of the client's beliefs. The therapist and client develop the activity to trial in daily life. For example, clients with the belief "No one likes me" might participate in an experiential activity where they engage with peers at a social setting. Clients who hold beliefs that they are "too tired" and "too helpless" to get out of bed are asked to challenge these cognitions by getting out of bed and engaging in an activity. The purpose of the exercise is to have the client test the validity of their thoughts by holding them up to real-world scenarios. Behavioral experiments, in addition to challenging thinking, also serve to decrease avoidance of places, situations, and settings, and thereby serve as a form of behavioral therapy. Other examples of behavioral experiments include confronting a friend or family member about an issue or conflict, practicing assertiveness in day-to-day life, public speaking, and engaging in volunteer work. As examples, several behavioral experiments were implemented with Mr. Doe, including challenging his beliefs of worthlessness and lack of purpose through doing volunteer work, having him pick up the phone to call his children rather than waiting for them to call, and saying yes when he received an invitation from family members. Role-plays and modeling can be used prior to executing the activity in the real world to help the client prepare and develop behavioral and cognitive skills (assertiveness, coping with strong emotions in the moment, etc.). After engaging in the exercise, clients are asked to reflect on their experience and its impact on their beliefs using a journal or log. Because real-world experiments are uncontrolled and may entail negative outcomes, the therapist and client should discuss these possibilities ahead of time and debrief as needed. For a detailed description and additional examples, please refer to Bennett-Levy et al.[90]

Sessions 13–15: Around Session 13, the Five-Column Dysfunctional Thought Record is introduced. The Five-Column Dysfunctional Thought Record includes the Three-Column Dysfunctional Thought record plus 2 additional columns for an alternative response and emotional consequences (Table 4.8). The Five-Column Dysfunctional Thought Record is used once the client has demonstrated a good understanding of the 3-column thought record and is readily able to identify and describe negative thinking patterns. It is recommended that the therapist work through 1–2 5-column worksheets before assigning one for practice. Below we list a sample Five-Column Dysfunctional Thought Record for Mr. Doe.

The therapist will assign the completion of one Five-Column Dysfunctional Thought Record per day between sessions, which will be reviewed and discussed at next session. At this point in therapy, challenging NATs in session should be very collaborative, with the therapist and client working together to review the past week's stressors and challenging thoughts together. Sessions 13–15 include reviewing the client's Five-Column Dysfunctional Thought Record for each week and engaging in Socratic dialogue.

Taking a look at Mr. Doe's Five-Column Dysfunctional Thought Record, it is clear that he was able to identify alternate beliefs that lessened the emotional toll of the situation. In session, the therapist reviewed several thought records from the previous week. Cognitive strategies used were aimed at increasing self-compassion and decreasing all-or-nothing thinking ("I didn't do

Table 4.8 Five-Column Dysfunctional Thought Record

What happened?	What did you tell yourself? (Rate on a 0–100 scale)	What emotion(s) or bodily responses did you experience? (Rate on a 0–100 scale)	Alternative response (what can you say or do that will be more helpful?)	Emotion Rate on a 0–100 scale
I did not get to the store as planned	I am stupid (100%) I am a failure (100%)	Sluggish (90%) Hopeless (90%) Depressed (100%) Bored (90%)	Just because I didn't go to the store earlier, doesn't mean the day is shot.	Sluggish (50%) Hopeless (40%) Depressed (50%) Bored (80%)
				Go back and rerate your original belief from 0–100.
			Sometimes my depression seems to "take over," but I know I am human and I have encountered this before.	
			I have been trying my best. Today does not reflect the entirety of the week.	I am stupid (40%) I am a failure (30%)

this, so I am a failure"). Through the review of several thought records, over the course of 2–3 weeks, Mr. Doe became more adept at recognizing his thought patterns and combating them. Eventually, he took more of the lead in session, challenging his own thoughts in real-time.

Modifying Core Beliefs (optional – add an additional ~4–5 sessions). Modifying at the level of core beliefs is necessary at times, usually in cases of chronic symptoms and/or personality features.[92] The need for modification at the level of core beliefs depends on the client's schema structure. For some clients, work at the level of situational dysfunctional thoughts (NATs) will suffice to shift thinking over a relatively short period of time. In these individuals, alternative schemas of themselves, others, and the world can be assessed as symptoms lift. However, for clients with chronic symptomatology, their schema structure is characterized by an absence of alternate healthy schemas; rather, they have enduring maladaptive schemas, and modification at a deeper cognitive level is required in order to develop new, healthier schemas.[93] Clinicians are advised to review James and Barton for a detailed review of this topic.[92]

As noted above, core beliefs refer to rigidly held and overgeneralized beliefs about the self, others, and the world. Returning to the cognitive model of psychopathology, the activation of core beliefs triggers a cascade of information processing biases affecting the onset and maintenance of psychopathology. For this reason, leaving core beliefs undisturbed creates vulnerability for future episodes of psychopathology. In addition, while many clients will experience symptom relief through challenging their NATs, many will experience the same thought, over and over again, if core beliefs are not targeted. Core beliefs originate from a deeper level of cognitive processing; thus, additional techniques are required for identification and modification. While a detailed description of core belief modification is beyond the scope of this chapter, we summarize the most commonly used therapeutic techniques. For an in-depth tutorial, we refer readers to James and Barton (2002); Padesky (1994).

Identifying Core Beliefs. Core beliefs may be obvious based on the client's verbalization. For example, Mr. Doe's underlying core beliefs were readily apparent through his verbalizations early on in therapy. However, many clients will not yet be able to verbalize core beliefs. Observing repeated and persistent NATs that cluster around a central theme (e.g., unlovable, worthless, failure, danger, etc.) often helps the therapist detect dysfunctional core beliefs. For instance, Ms. Jones voiced frequent NATs related to feeling rejected by her family members ("No one cares about me," "I am a burden on others," "I have nothing left to contribute"). Her NATs arose in situations in which she perceived a slight from family members, such as missing a phone call, detecting a lack of excitement when they visited her, and failing to ask about her day when they did visit. Applying the thought-challenging techniques described above helped her cope better in situations in which these beliefs were activated, but she continued to experience frequent activation of these core beliefs. In addition, her emotional response to the event appeared out of proportion to the situation, with tearfulness and withdrawal above what would be expected when considering the situational antecedent. When core beliefs are activated, they generally are affect-laden, as they draw from historical pain, not just the present situation. Thus, NATs that evoke a disproportionate level of affect and emotional response often indicate the manifestation of a core belief. Attending to content that evokes strong affect will likely uncover core beliefs.

To guide identification, the **Downward Arrow Technique** is used.[83,94] This technique involves using Socratic dialogue to uncover the underlying core belief behind a negative automatic thought. The exercise involves questioning the client about the meaning he or she has attached to a particular negative automatic thought. Eventually, layers are stripped away to reveal the underlying core belief, which is apparent because no further meaning can be derived.

Additional techniques to access schemas can be found in Padesky (1994), including the use of Socratic questioning to access self, other, and world schemas, and sentence completion exercises.

After identifying core beliefs, several techniques can be used to challenge them. First, all of the cognitive challenging techniques described above may be appropriate, in particular, weighing the evidence and challenging the utility of the belief. Specifying the source of the message and at what period in time the message developed can also be useful. Core belief worksheets can help the client test the veracity of unhelpful core beliefs in daily life.[84]

In the case of Mr. John Doe, his core belief of worthlessness developed from early messages from his father. Clarifying the source of the message (father), age and context (in childhood, when his father was intoxicated), and examining the veracity of this message across the life course (at age 10, age 20, age 30, etc.) produced flexibility in responding and greater perspective taking when this core belief was triggered and eventually reduced the frequency and intensity of activation altogether, because he was focused more on the present rather than drawing upon "old messages" from the past. Sample worksheets that take a developmental approach in challenging core beliefs can be found in Gallagher-Thompson and Thompson.[85]

As the old core belief is identified, the therapist helps the client identify and incorporate evidence to support a new healthier core belief. This typically occurs through work outside

Table 4.9 Example Positive Data Log

New belief: I have worth	
Day	**Evidence for**
Monday	I went to my volunteer job. People were happy to see me.
Tuesday	I received a call from my son. I disclosed I had been feeling down today, and he listened and told me he loved me.
Wednesday	I took a walk around my apartment complex. A neighbor smiled and said hello and asked how I was doing.
Thursday	I reflected on my role as a father. I did my best. I cared for them and gave them a better life than I had.
Friday	I made it to the store, even though my "depression" told me not to leave the house.

of the therapy session, through the use of logs and monitoring sheets to help the client incorporate evidence to support the new core belief. Examples include the Positive Data Log.[95] The Positive Data Log instructs the client to track evidence supporting a new core belief. For instance, in the case of Mr. John Doe, he began tracking evidence in his day-to-day life supporting his self-worth. (See Appendix C for a blank copy.)

Behavioral experiments can also be applied to challenge unhelpful core beliefs as well as conditional beliefs. Below we describe the two most common behavioral experiments. The goal of the exercise is to begin challenging long-held maladaptive schemas and facilitate the adoption of healthier schemas. Behavioral experiments, in addition to Socratic dialogue, are essential for this change to occur.

As If is a basic, yet effective, behavioral experiment that has the client act "as if" a new healthier schema is in place. For example, Mr. Doe was asked to suspend his belief that he had no inherent worth or lovability and act "as if" he did. This entailed taking care of himself (feeding himself regular meals, getting exercise, taking regular showers) and picking up and making phone calls. He also acted "as if" by applying assertiveness skills to seek volunteer work and communicating more effectively with his daughter and son about his feelings concerning their relationships. When testing out "as if," it's important to frame the exercise as an experiment ("We're going to test behaving 'as if' and then observe the effects"). It can be useful to pick one activity at a time that adopts and tests out the new core belief, for example, starting with more self-care activities as a first step and then creating a second experiment that involves interpersonal relationship and communication skills.

Continuum Technique. The continuum technique involves processing dichotomous core beliefs using continuous properties, with the goal of enhancing cognitive flexibility and enhancing more realistic and less negatively biased schemas.[92,93] The therapist and the client create a horizontal line from 0–100%, with 100% reflecting the opposite belief from the maladaptive core belief. For example, in the case of Mr. Doe, at 100% was the belief "Self-worth." Clients are instructed to provide an initial rating of where they fall currently. They are also asked to denote where other individuals either from their own life or in history fall along the line. As clients consider the full range of individuals anchored at various points along the line, the therapist uses Socratic dialogue to question clients' place on the line. The exercise assists clients in gaining perspective on ways they may be

Table 4.10 Example Criteria Continua for Self-Worth[93]

Self-Worth:		
0% X Mr. Doe's rating pre-exercise	X Mr. Doe's rating after exercise	100%
Always alone		Someone loving and caring; is always present
Never experiences positive emotions		Always happy
Does nothing productive ever		Always engaged in a productive task
Gives nothing to the world or to others		Constantly giving to others and the world

judging themselves harshly. For example, Mr. Doe initially placed himself at 10% worth. As the exercise proceeded, he placed several family members at one hundred percent. He had difficulty perceiving others as having lower worth, but with continued questioning placed corrupt political figures, a bully from the military, and an old boss as lower mid-range on the continuum. After placing others on the line, he was asked again to consider his position and moved himself to above 40%, reflecting a significant increase in his perception of worth. Another useful version of the continuum technique involves an exercise called **criteria continua**, which provides behavioral descriptions of schematic content. For example, Mr. Doe was asked to provide behavioral descriptions of having self-worth at 0% and 100% anchors. This technique helps operationalize what is meant by "worth" to clients and facilitates use of behavioral terms that can foster more realistic and balanced thinking.

Sessions 16–18: Feeling Skills

Feeling skills provides a set of tools that reduce anxiety and depressive rumination by helping clients gain awareness of their stress and tension levels and develop relaxation strategies. Feeling skills can also "slow down" thinking during highly stressful times in order to provide time to problem-solve. In this section, we provide a basic overview of the most common feeling skills used in CBT. The order of skills is flexible between Sessions 16 and 18 but generally begins with psychoeducation followed by teaching clients how to use the tension diary and relaxation strategies.

Relaxation Training. Relaxation training is a 2-step process. In the first step, clients build awareness of the triggers to their anxiety and stress through the use of a tension diary (Appendix D). The tension diary has clients track on a daily basis their level of tension (1–10), source of stress, and experience of stress. The second step involves creating a relaxation practice. The client is taught a menu of relaxation strategies, which may include diaphragmatic breathing, progressive muscle relaxation, guided imagery, music, and exercise, among others. Clients are advised to practice relaxation one time per day, for 5–30 minutes at a time or more.

Diaphragmatic Breathing. Breathing retraining teaches clients about the connection between breathing and stress responses. Most patients take to this exercise easily. It involves short psychoeducation about how breathing can affect anxiety levels. The therapist describes how, when stressed or anxious, we tend to take shallow breaths, which can increase the body's stress response. As an example, clients may take a few shallow, quick breaths to observe their effect on the level of anxiety they are experiencing. Clients are then shown how to take full, deep breaths, expanding their diaphragms and then exhaling out through their mouths (or noses). Each inhalation and exhalation should take three to four seconds, although this may vary based on clients' physical health status. Clients can evoke a greater relaxation response by pairing paced breathing with music, a quiet room or environment, guided imagery, or aromatherapy.

Mr. Doe applied paced breathing on a regular basis, typically in the mornings, as he started his day. He tracked his tension scores before and after paced breathing and found the short exercise helpful at reducing rumination and anxiety in the morning. He also applied the exercise at night, when he tended to worry more.

Progressive Muscle Relaxation (PMR). Progressive muscle relaxation is an exercise that involves tensing and relaxing various muscle groups.[96] The goal is for clients to begin recognizing where they hold tension throughout their bodies and how to release it. As they gain awareness of where in the body they tend to hold tension, they come to recognize the difference between tensed and relaxed muscle states. For older adults who may not be able to engage in the tensing portion of PMR, passive PMR is available, which involves systematically relaxing muscle groups without using the tensing component.[97] Several PMR scripts are freely available online.

Progressive muscle relaxation was used in session with Mr. Doe, and he was provided a recording of PMR to take home. He practiced PMR at least one time per week and found it helpful in reducing overall tension. He also applied it when he felt himself ruminating on the loss of his wife.

Guided Imagery. Guided imagery involves bringing to one's mind a relaxing, calming, and tranquil scene either from memory or created for the exercise. To guide the exercise, clinicians can access scripts online, such as beach scenes, or a script can be created in session based on the client's memory. When practicing guided imagery, the client is instructed to focus, accessing the scene with all five senses. Many other guided imagery scripts are available for free online.

Sessions 19–20: Termination and Relapse Prevention. When preparing for treatment termination, it is helpful to complete several tasks, which ideally begin 2–3 sessions prior to termination. For some clients, it can be helpful to spread out the last few sessions of therapy, to facilitate adjustment and trialing skills without weekly contact. For others, it can be useful to have a booster session scheduled one or two months after treatment termination. As noted at the beginning of the therapy, clients should be socialized at the beginning of therapy concerning the time-limited nature of treatment so they are not surprised when discussions about treatment termination arise.

In preparation for treatment termination, several tasks are required. First, it is prudent to process the relationship prior to termination. Clients will vary on how attached or reluctant they are to terminate therapy; therefore, it is important to process the client's feeling about ending the relationship. The therapist may share his or her own experience working with the client and what was learned from their work together. This allows for a transparent dialogue about the potential meaning and value of the therapeutic relationship itself and the processing of any emotional reactions or beliefs associated with termination of the therapeutic relationship. Second, reassessment of symptoms is needed as well as a review of the progress made at meeting initial therapy goals. Clients may find it rewarding to visualize the change in their symptoms over time, through use of a simple line graph demonstrating change. When reviewing therapy goals, the therapist will return to measurable indices of success (described at the beginning of the chapter), to be reviewed with the client. In addition, the client's subjective experience of progress, growth, and improvement are also discussed and documented. Third, the client and therapist will work together to create a relapse prevention plan. Relapse prevention plans are personalized and based on the patient's presenting problem. They typically include warning signs of relapse, how to identify situations and stressors ahead of time that may affect relapse, review of key coping skills and when to use them, and when to reach out for support and professional help.

Below we present a sample relapse prevention plan for Mr. Doe. His primary warning signs were identified, along with anticipated stressors, and main ways of coping with mood, anxiety, and stress symptoms. He was provided a copy of his relapse prevention plan, along with a notebook of blank worksheets.

Conclusion of Mr. Doe's Case: At end of the session, Mr. Doe experienced a reduction in depression (PHQ-9 = 8) and anxiety symptoms (GAI = 6), and subjectively reported more awareness of his thinking patterns and a greater ability to challenge thoughts in real-time. He continued to use activity scheduling, particularly when he noted himself slipping into old patterns of withdrawing. He no longer expressed passive or active suicidal ideation

Table 4.11 Relapse Prevention Plan for Mr. John Doe

My warning signs
- Ruminate on loss of wife
- Disengage from activities, do not leave house
- Start feeling hopeless again

Anticipated stressors and situations
- Physical decline
- Holidays and anniversaries of life with wife

Main coping skills
- Activity monitoring form when I observe myself isolating
- When my thoughts get more negative, I will begin using the Five-Column Dysfunctional Thought Record
- I will keep practicing relaxation daily, which helps me feel more balanced and decreases rumination

If I need help
- Call my son or sister. I may or may not share how I am feeling at this point, but it helps to know they care.
- Call therapist for a booster session.
- If in a mental health crisis, present to local urgent care/emergency department, call 911, or call the national suicide prevention hotline.

and was more active in his community through volunteer work. He talked to his family more and was in the process of moving closer to where they lived. While he missed his wife very much, he reported feeling less debilitated by grief and was able to experience more positive emotions day-to-day. He described having greater agency and empowerment, which was noted in his active participation in his relapse prevention plan. He was better able to recognize when core beliefs were activated and used a Positive Data Log when this occurred. He practiced diaphragmatic breathing in the mornings or when he felt more anxious.

Conclusions

Cognitive behavioral therapy is an effective, evidenced-based treatment for late-life psychiatric disorders and can be delivered in various modalities and settings. Providers take a collaborative stance focused on helping the client gain greater insight concerning unhelpful thinking and behavioral patterns and learn active strategies to cope with distress. Therapeutic change occurs through a combination of thinking and behavior modification. Cognitive behavioral therapy is appropriate for the majority of older adults, with some modifications being necessary when working with cognitively impaired clients.

Resources

Organizations Offering CBT Training

- **Beck Institute:** The Beck Institute offers a full program complete with online and in-person courses, and workshops that cover fundamental knowledge and skills as well as specialty areas (e.g., CBT for suicide prevention, CBT for chronic pain and opioid use), although it lacks courses that provide instruction specific to working with older adults (https://beckinstitute.org/beck-learning-path/). When implementing a new treatment, supervision or consultation from a trained licensed practitioner is imperative, and the Beck Institute offers this service.
- **Association for Behavioral and Cognitive Therapies (ABCT):** The ABCT website contains a range of training resources, including free videos, webcasts, and podcasts, as well as a list of relevant self-help books, treatment manuals, and training videos (www.abct.org/Resources/?m=mResources&fa=Videos).
- **American Psychological Association's Continuing Education Programs in Psychology:** APA offers several continuing education programs on CBT for specific clinical presentations (e.g., complicated depression, suicidal patients) and older adults (e.g., "Treatment of late-life depression, anxiety, trauma, and substance abuse") (www.apa.org/education/ce/index.aspx).
- **University of East Anglia:** The University of East Anglia offers a three-week online course titled "CBT with Older People," which can be found on the Future Learn website (www.futurelearn.com/courses/cbt-older-people).
- **The American Institute for Cognitive Therapy:** The website contains a list of recommended readings, helpful links to blog posts and sample chapters, and podcasts and YouTube videos on CBT. The American Institute for Cognitive Therapy also offers workshops, supervision, and consultation (https://cognitivetherapynyc.com/Default.aspx).

Books, Manuals, and Other Readings

- *Cognitive Behavior Therapy with Older Adults: Innovations Across Care Settings* by Sorocco & Lauderdale (2011)
- *CBT For Older People: An Introduction* by Laidlaw (2015)
- *Handbook of Behavioral and Cognitive Therapies with Older Adults* by Gallagher-Thompson, Steffen, and Thompson (2008)
- *Cognitive Behaviour Therapy with Older People* by Laidlaw, Thompson, Dick-Siskin, and Gallagher-Thompson (2003)
- *A Clinician's Guide to CBT with Older People* by Laidlaw, Kishita, and Chellingsworth (2016) (www.uea.ac.uk/documents/246046/8314842/FINAL+VERSION+CBT+WITH+OLDER+PEOPLE.pdf/542cb385-aa69-4df3-906d-c72363f36046)
- *A Clinician's Guide to Low Intensity CBT with Older People* by Chellingsworth, Kishita, & Laidlaw (2016) (www.uea.ac.uk/documents/246046/8314842/LICBT_BOOKLET_FINAL_JAN16.pdf/48f28e80-dc02-45b6-91cd-c628d36e8bca)
- Treatments That Work Series
  - *Treating Late-Life Depression: A Cognitive-Behavioral Therapy Approach* (2009)
  - *A Cognitive-Behavioral Approach to the Beginning of the End of Life* (2008)

References

1. Laidlaw K, Thompson LW, Dick-Siskin L, Gallagher-Thompson D. *Cognitive behaviour therapy with older people.* New York: John Wiley & Sons; 2003. p. xvi, 215.

2. Laidlaw K. An empirical review of cognitive therapy for late life depression: does research evidence suggest adaptations are necessary for cognitive therapy with older adults? *Clin Psychol Psychother.* 2001;8(1):1–14.

3. Karlin BE. Cognitive behavioral therapy with older adults. In: Lauderdale KHSS, editor. *Cognitive behavior therapy with older adults: innovations across care settings.* New York: Springer; 2011. p. 1–28.

4. Laidlaw K, McAlpine S. Cognitive behaviour therapy: how is it different with older people? *J Ration Emot Cogn Behav Ther.* 2008;26(4):250–262.

5. Beck AT. *Depression: clinical, experimental, and theoretical aspects.* New York: Hoeber Medical Division, Harper & Row; 1967.

6. Lewinsohn PM, Sullivan JM, Grosscup SJ. Changing reinforcing events: an approach to the treatment of depression. *Psychotherapy: Theory, Research & Practice.* 1980;17(3):322–334.

7. Clark DA, Beck AT. *Cognitive therapy of anxiety disorders: science and practice.* New York: Guilford Press; 2010. p. ix, 628.

8. Wright JH, Beck AT. Cognitive therapy of depression: theory and practice. *Psychiatric Services.* 1983;34(12):1119–1127.

9. Gould RL, Coulson MC, Howard RJ. Cognitive behavioral therapy for depression in older people: a meta-analysis and meta-regression of randomized controlled trials. *Journal Am Geriatr Soc.* 2012;60(10):1817–1830.

10. Pinquart M, Duberstein P, Lyness J. Effects of psychotherapy and other behavioral interventions on clinically depressed older adults: a meta-analysis. *Aging Ment Health.* 2007;11(6):645–657.

11. Peng X, Huang C, Chen L, Lu Z. Cognitive behavioural therapy and reminiscence techniques for the treatment of depression in the elderly: a systematic review. *Journal of International Medical Research.* 2009;37(4):975–982.

12. Wilson K, Mottram PG, Vassilas C. Psychotherapeutic treatments for older depressed people. *Cochrane database of systematic reviews.* 2008(1): CD004853.

13. Gould RL, Coulson MC, Howard RJ. Efficacy of cognitive behavioral therapy for anxiety disorders in older people: a meta-analysis and meta-regression of randomized controlled trials. *J Am Geriatr Soc.* 2012;60(2):218–229.

14. Hall J, Kellett S, Berrios R, Bains MK, Scott S. Efficacy of cognitive behavioral therapy for generalized anxiety disorder in older adults: systematic review, meta-analysis, and meta-regression. *American J of Geriatr Psychiatry.* 2016;24(11): 1063–1073.

15. Hendriks G, Oude Voshaar R, Keijsers G, Hoogduin C, Van Balkom A. Cognitive-behavioural therapy for late-life anxiety disorders: a systematic review and meta-analysis. *Acta Psychiatr Scand.* 2008;117 (6):403–411.

16. Granholm E, McQuaid JR, McClure FS, et al. Randomized controlled trial of cognitive behavioral social skills training for older people with schizophrenia: 12-month follow-up. *J Clin Psychiatry.* 2007;68 (5):730–737.

17. Mueser KT, Deavers F, Penn DL, Cassisi JE. Psychosocial treatments for schizophrenia. *Annual review of clinical psychology.* 2013;9:465–497.

18. Reiser R, Reddy S, Parkins MM, Thompson LW, Gallagher-Thompson D. Psychosocial treatment of bipolar disorder in older adults. *Cognitive Behavior Therapy with Older Adults.* 2011:65.

19. Swartz HA, Swanson J. Psychotherapy for bipolar disorder in adults: a review of the evidence. *Focus.* 2014;12(3):251–266.

20. Miklowitz DJ, Otto MW, Frank E, et al. Psychosocial treatments for bipolar depression: a 1-year randomized trial from the Systematic Treatment Enhancement Program. *Arch Gen Psychiatry.* 2007;64 (4):419–426.

21. Clapp JD, Beck JG. Treatment of PTSD in older adults: do cognitive-behavioral interventions remain viable? *Cogn Behav Pract.* 2012;19(1):126–135.

22. Cook JM, McCarthy E, Thorp SR. Older adults with PTSD: brief state of research and evidence-based psychotherapy case illustration. *Am J Geriatr Psychiatry.* 2017;25(5):522–530.

23. Thorp SR, Stein MB, Jeste DV, Patterson TL, Wetherell JL. Prolonged exposure therapy for older veterans with posttraumatic stress disorder: a pilot study. *Am J Geriatr Psychiatry.* 2012;20 (3):276–280.

24. McCurry SM, Logsdon RG, Teri L, Vitiello MV. Evidence-based psychological treatments for insomnia in older adults. *Psychol Aging.* 2007;22(1):18.

25. Montgomery P, Dennis JA. Cognitive behavioural interventions for sleep problems in adults aged 60+. *Cochrane database of systematic reviews.* 2003(1).

26. Irwin MR, Cole JC, Nicassio PM. Comparative meta-analysis of behavioral interventions for insomnia and their efficacy in middle-aged adults and in older adults 55+ years of age. *Health Psychology.* 2006;25(1):3.

27. Bélanger L, LeBlanc M, Morin CM. Cognitive behavioral therapy for insomnia in older adults. *Cognitive and Behavioral Practice.* 2012;19(1):101–115.

28. Ehde DM, Dillworth TM, Turner JA. Cognitive-behavioral therapy for individuals with chronic pain: efficacy, innovations, and directions for research. *American Psychologist.* 2014;69(2):153.

29. Lunde L-H, Nordhus IH, Pallesen S. The effectiveness of cognitive and behavioural treatment of chronic pain in the elderly: a quantitative review. *J Clin Psychol Medical Settings.* 2009;16(3):254–262.

30. Nicholas MK, Asghari A, Blyth FM, et al. Self-management intervention for chronic pain in older adults: a randomised controlled trial. *PAIN.* 2013;154 (6):824–835.

31. Hummel SB, Van Lankveld JJ, Oldenburg HS, et al. Efficacy of internet-based cognitive behavioral therapy in improving sexual functioning of breast cancer survivors: results of a randomized controlled trial. *J Clin Oncol.* 2017;35 (12):1328–1340.

32. Kunik M, Veazey C, Cully J, et al. COPD education and cognitive behavioral therapy

group treatment for clinically significant symptoms of depression and anxiety in COPD patients: a randomized controlled trial. *Psychological Medicine*. 2008;38 (3):385–396.

33. Wetherell JL, Gatz M, Craske MG. Treatment of generalized anxiety disorder in older adults. *J Consult Clin Psychol*. 2003;71(1):31.

34. Wuthrich V, Rapee R, Kangas M, Perini S. Randomized controlled trial of group cognitive behavioral therapy compared to a discussion group for co-morbid anxiety and depression in older adults. *Psychological Medicine*. 2016;46 (4):785–795.

35. Zijlstra GR, Van Haastregt JC, Ambergen T, et al. Effects of a multicomponent cognitive behavioral group intervention on fear of falling and activity avoidance in community-dwelling older adults: results of a randomized controlled trial. *J Am Geriatr Soc*. 2009;57(11):2020–2028.

36. Dear BF, Zou JB, Ali S, et al. Clinical and cost-effectiveness of therapist-guided internet-delivered cognitive behavior therapy for older adults with symptoms of anxiety: a randomized controlled trial. *Behavior Therapy*. 2015;46(2):206–217.

37. O'moore KA, Newby JM, Andrews G, et al. Internet cognitive–behavioral therapy for depression in older adults with knee osteoarthritis: a randomized controlled trial. *Arthritis Care & Research*. 2018;70 (1):61–70.

38. Spek V, Cuijpers P, Nyklíček I, et al. One-year follow-up results of a randomized controlled clinical trial on internet-based cognitive behavioural therapy for subthreshold depression in people over 50 years. *Psychological Medicine*. 2008;38 (5):635–639.

39. Titov N, Dear BF, Ali S, et al. Clinical and cost-effectiveness of therapist-guided internet-delivered cognitive behavior therapy for older adults with symptoms of depression: a randomized controlled trial. *Behavior Therapy*. 2015;46(2):193–205.

40. Lichstein KL, Scogin F, Thomas SJ, et al. Telehealth cognitive behavior therapy for

co-occurring insomnia and depression symptoms in older adults. *J Clin Psychol*. 2013;69(10):1056–1065.

41. Rybarczyk B, Lopez M, Schelble K, Stepanski E. Home-based video CBT for comorbid geriatric insomnia: a pilot study using secondary data analyses. *Behav Sleep Med*. 2005;3(3):158–175.

42. Brenes GA, Danhauer SC, Lyles MF, Hogan PE, Miller ME. Telephone-delivered cognitive behavioral therapy and telephone-delivered nondirective supportive therapy for rural older adults with generalized anxiety disorder: a randomized clinical trial. *JAMA Psychiatry*. 2015;72(10):1012–1020.

43. Hyer L, Yeager CA, Hilton N, Sacks A. Group, individual, and staff therapy: an efficient and effective cognitive behavioral therapy in long-term care. *Am J Alzheimers Dis Other Demen*. 2009;23(6):528–539.

44. Cully JA, Stanley MA, Petersen NJ, et al. Delivery of brief cognitive behavioral therapy for medically ill patients in primary care: a pragmatic randomized clinical trial. *J Gen Intern Med*. 2017;32(9):1014–1024.

45. Holvast F, Massoudi B, Voshaar RCO, Verhaak PF. Non-pharmacological treatment for depressed older patients in primary care: a systematic review and meta-analysis. *PloS One*. 2017;12(9): e0184666.

46. DiNapoli EA, Pierpaoli CM, Shah A, Yang X, Scogin F. Effects of home-delivered cognitive behavioral therapy (CBT) for depression on anxiety symptoms among rural, *ethnically diverse older adults*. *Clinical Gerontologist*. 2017;40(3):181–190.

47. Cully JA, Stanley MA, Deswal A, et al. Cognitive-behavioral therapy for chronic cardiopulmonary conditions: preliminary outcomes from an open trial. *Primary Care Companion to the Journal of Clinical Psychiatry*. 2010;12(4).

48. Freedland KE, Carney RM, Rich MW, Steinmeyer BC, Rubin EH. Cognitive behavior therapy for depression and self-care in heart failure patients: a randomized clinical trial. *JAMA Intern Med*. 2015;175 (11):1773–1782.

49. Jeyanantham K, Kotecha D, Thanki D, Dekker R, Lane DA. Effects of cognitive behavioural therapy for depression in heart failure patients: a systematic review and meta-analysis. *Heart Failure Rev.* 2017;22 (6):731–741.

50. Calleo JS, Amspoker AB, Sarwar AI, et al. A pilot study of a cognitive-behavioral treatment for anxiety and depression in patients with Parkinson disease. *J Geriatr Psychiatry Neurol.* 2015;28(3):210–217.

51. Egan SJ, Laidlaw K, Starkstein S. Cognitive behaviour therapy for depression and anxiety in Parkinson's disease. *J Parkinsons Dis.* 2015;5(3):443–451.

52. Broomfield NM, Laidlaw K, Hickabottom E, et al. Post-stroke depression: the case for augmented, individually tailored cognitive behavioural therapy. *Clinical Psychology and Psychotherapy.* 2011;18(3):202–217.

53. Kneebone II. A framework to support cognitive behavior therapy for emotional disorder after stroke. *Cogn Behav Pract.* 2016;23(1):99–109.

54. Scogin F, Morthland M, Kaufman A, et al. Improving quality of life in diverse rural older adults: a randomized trial of a psychological treatment. *Psychol Aging.* 2007;22(4):657.

55. Stanley MA, Wilson N, Shrestha S, et al. Calmer Life: a culturally tailored intervention for anxiety in underserved older adults. *American J Geriatr Psychiatry.* 2016;24(8):648–658.

56. Kraus CA, Seignourel P, Balasubramanyam V, et al. Cognitive-behavioral treatment for anxiety in patients with dementia: two case studies. *J Psychiatr Pract.* 2008;14(3):186.

57. Orgeta V, Qazi A, Spector A, Orrell M. Psychological treatments for depression and anxiety in dementia and mild cognitive impairment: systematic review and meta-analysis. *BJPsych.* 2015;207(4):293–298.

58. Snow AL, Powers D, Liles D. Cognitive-behavioral therapy for long-term care patients with dementia. *Geropsychological Interventions in Long-Term Care.* 2006:265–283.

59. Spector A, Charlesworth G, King M, et al. Cognitive-behavioural therapy for anxiety in dementia: pilot randomised controlled trial. *BJPsych.* 2015;206(6):509–516.

60. Stanley MA, Calleo J, Bush AL, et al. The Peaceful Mind program: a pilot test of a cognitive-behavioral therapy-based intervention for anxious patients with Dementia. *Am J Geriatr Psychiatry.* 2013;21 (7):696–708.

61. Teri L, Gallagher-Thompson D. Cognitive-behavioral interventions for treatment of depression in Alzheimer's patients. *Gerontologist.* 1991;31(3):413–416.

62. Hundt NE, Amspoker AB, Kraus-Schuman C, et al. Predictors of CBT outcome in older adults with GAD. *J Anxiety Disord.* 2014;28(8):845–850.

63. Wetherell JL, Hopko DR, Diefenbach GJ, et al. Cognitive-behavioral therapy for late-life generalized anxiety disorder: Who gets better? *Behavior Therapy.* 2005;36 (2):147–156.

64. Kishita N, Laidlaw K. Cognitive behaviour therapy for generalized anxiety disorder: is CBT equally efficacious in adults of working age and older adults? *Clin Psychol Rev.* 2017;52:124–136.

65. Conti EC, Barrera TL, Amspoker AB, et al. Predictors of outcomes for older adults participating in Calmer Life, a culturally tailored intervention for anxiety. *Clinical Gerontol.* 2017;40(3):172–180.

66. Marquett RM, Thompson LW, Reiser RP, et al. Psychosocial predictors of treatment response to cognitive-behavior therapy for late-life depression: an exploratory study. *Aging Ment Health.* 2013;17 (7):830–838.

67. Mohlman J, Gorenstein EE, Kleber M, et al. Standard and enhanced cognitive-behavior therapy for late-life generalized anxiety disorder: two pilot investigations. *Am J Geriatr Psychiatry.* 2003;11(1):24–32.

68. Kazantzis N, Pachana NA, Secker DL. Cognitive behavioral therapy for older adults: practical guidelines for the use of homework assignments. *Cogn Behav Pract.* 2003;10(4):324–332.

69. Kroenke K, Spitzer RL, Williams JB, Löwe B. The patient health questionnaire somatic, anxiety, and depressive symptom

scales: a systematic review. *Gen Hosp Psychiatry*. 2010;32(4):345–359.

70. Yesavage JA, Sheikh JI. 9/Geriatric depression scale (GDS) recent evidence and development of a shorter version. *Clinical Gerontologist*. 1986;5(1–2):165–173.

71. Pachana NA, Byrne GJ, Siddle H, et al. Development and validation of the Geriatric Anxiety Inventory. *Int Psychogeriatr*. 2007;19(1):103–114.

72. Covin R, Dozois DJ, Ogniewicz A, Seeds PM. Measuring cognitive errors: Initial development of the Cognitive Distortions Scale (CDS). *Int J Cogn Ther*. 2011;4 (3):297–322.

73. Laidlaw K, Thompson LW, Gallagher-Thompson D. Comprehensive conceptualization of cognitive behaviour therapy for late life depression. *Behav Cogn Psychother*. 2004;32(4):389–399.

74. Conti E, Arnspiger C, Uriate J, Kraus-Schuman C, Batiste, M. 2016. Retrieved from: www.mirecc.va.gov/VISN16/docs/Safety_Planning_for_Older_Adults_Manual.pdf

75. Beck AT. Cognitive models of depression. *J Cogn Psychother*. 1987;1(1):5–37.

76. Wenzel, A, Dobson, KS, Hays, PA. *Cognitive behavioral therapy techniques and strategies*. American Psychological Association; 2016.

77. Neumann PJ, Araki SS, Gutterman EM. The use of proxy respondents in studies of older adults: lessons, challenges, and opportunities. *J Am Geriatr Soc*. 2000;48 (12):1646–1654.

78. Wenzel A. *Innovations in cognitive behavioral therapy: strategic interventions for creative practice*: New York: Routledge; 2017.

79. MacPhillamy DJ, Lewinsohn PM. The pleasant events schedule: studies on reliability, validity, and scale intercorrelation. *J Consult Clin Psychol*. 1982;50(3):363.

80. Rider K, Gallagher-Thompson D, Thompson L. California older person's pleasant events schedule: manual. 2004;14:2006. *Retrieved from:* http://med.stanford.edu/oafc/coppes.html

81. Nezu AM, Nezu CM, Lombardo ER. *Cognitive-behavioral case formulation and treatment design: a problem-solving approach*: New York: Springer; 2004.

82. Overholser JC. Guided discovery. *J Contemp Psychother*. 2013;43(2):73–82.

83. Beck AT, Rush AJ, Shaw Bf, Emery G. *Cognitive therapy of depression*. New York: Guilford Press; 1979.

84. Beck AT, Dozois DJ. Cognitive therapy: current status and future directions. *Annu Rev Med*. 2011;62:397–409.

85. Gallagher-Thompson D, Thompson LW. *Treating late life depression: a cognitive-behavioral therapy approach, therapist guide*. New York: Oxford University Press; 2009.

86. Hofmann SG, Asmundson GJ. Acceptance and mindfulness-based therapy: new wave or old hat? *Clin Psychol Rev*. 2008;28 (1):1–16.

87. MacBeth A, Gumley A. Exploring compassion: a meta-analysis of the association between self-compassion and psychopathology. *Clin Psychol Rev* 2012;32 (6):545–552.

88. Ruiz FJ. A review of Acceptance and Commitment Therapy (ACT) empirical evidence: correlational, experimental psychopathology, component and outcome studies. *International Journal of Psychology and Psychological Therapy*. 2010;10(1).

89. Neff KD, Kirkpatrick KL, Rude SS. Self-compassion and adaptive psychological functioning. *J Res Pers*. 2007;41 (1):139–154.

90. Bennett-Levy J, Westbrook D, Fennell M, et al. Behavioural experiments: historical and conceptual underpinnings. *Oxford Guide to Behavioural Experiments in Cognitive Therapy*. 2004:1–20.

91. Rutter J, Friedberg R. Guidelines for the effective use of Socratic dialogue in cognitive therapy. *Innovations in Clinical Practice: A Source Book*. 1999;17:481–490.

92. James IA, Barton S. Changing core beliefs with the continuum technique. *Behav Cogn Psychother*. 2004;32(4):431–442.

93. Padesky CA. Schema change processes in cognitive therapy. *Clin Psychol Psychother.* 1994;1(5):267–278.

94. Burns D. *Feeling good: the new mood therapy.* New York: William Morrow; 1980.

95. Dobson D, Dobson KS. *Evidence-based practice of cognitive-behavioral therapy.* New York: Guilford Press; 2018.

96. Bernstein DA, Borkovec TD, Hazlett-Stevens H. *New directions in progressive relaxation training: a guidebook for helping professionals.* Westport, CT: Greenwood; 2000.

97. Feldman G, Greeson J, Senville J. Differential effects of mindful breathing, progressive muscle relaxation, and loving-kindness meditation on decentering and negative reactions to repetitive thoughts. *Behaviour Research and Therapy.* 2010;48 (10):1002–1011.

Appendix A What Is Cognitive Behavioral Therapy?

Cognitive Behavioral Therapy or CBT is a time-limited (16–20 sessions) treatment that is skill based and collaborative. We will work together to create therapy goals, create a plan for treatment, and learn skills to change your thinking and behavior patterns that cause distress in your life. The therapy will focus on your activity levels, as well as your interpretation of events in your life. We will do this by observing the connection between events, thoughts ("What I tell myself"), and your emotional (feeling), behavioral ("What did I do?"), and physiological response ("How does my body feel?"). Below we present the basic cognitive behavioral model. **Please practice completing one in the next week.**

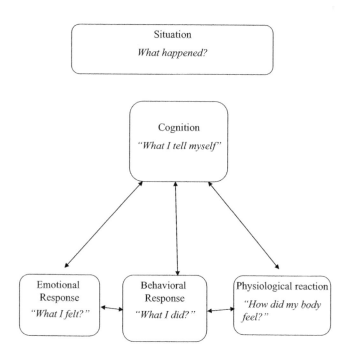

Appendix B Problem-Solving Worksheet

1. Problem: _____

2. Goal: _____

3. Solutions:

    Pros   Cons

4. Select a solution: _____

5. Evaluate
   consequences: _____
   _____
   _____

Appendix C Positive Data Log

New belief: I have worth	
Day	Evidence for
Monday	
Tuesday	
Wednesday	
Thursday	
Friday	

Appendix D Tension Diary

Rate your tension on a 0–10 scale (0 = least tense; 10 = most tense), where in the body you experience it, and situation.

Day	Monday	Tuesday	Wednesday	Thursday	Friday	Saturday	Sunday
Most tense #							
Where in the body?							
Situation							

Problem-Solving Therapy

Brenna N. Renn, Brittany A. Mosser, and Patrick J. Raue

Introduction

Problem-solving therapy (PST) is an evidence-based psychotherapy for depression with particularly robust evidence for use among older adults. The primary intervention of PST is teaching people to deal more effectively with their difficulties, or problems, in order to reduce psychopathology and enhance functioning and well-being. Problem-solving therapy was first developed in the 1970s as an extension of behavior modification that involved cognitive processes to arrive at possible solutions to problems; the intervention has been refined and modified in the ensuing decades.[1,2] A large body of scientific evidence supports PST as an effective intervention for depression; however, more recent applications discussed herein use PST to alleviate other aging-related difficulties, including chronic disease, cognitive impairment (CI), and disability. All variations of PST share the same core features, including an emphasis on specifying the problem, setting goals, and creating action plans to achieve those goals.

We present the theoretical framework of PST and review a typical course of treatment, which is focused on addressing problems in the context of depressive symptoms, with an emphasis on setting goals and creating action plans to achieve those goals. We will use the case of Mrs. Rodriguez to illustrate a course of PST with a 69-year-old woman with depression and mild CI secondary to Parkinson's disease.

Description of the Approach

Theoretical Framework

Problem-solving therapy is a skills-based approach that treats depression by teaching patients how to systematically solve problems, set feasible goals, and create specific action plans to achieve those goals, with the aim of reducing symptomatology and maximizing quality of life.[1,2] "Problems" are any situation in which there is a discrepancy between the present and desired conditions, and in which an immediate solution is not apparent. Problem-solving is the process by which a person attempts to effectively resolve, adapt, or cope with such situations. We routinely engage in problem-solving as we go about many of our daily activities, such as deciding on how to prioritize competing demands at home and work, starting an exercise routine, or resolving a disagreement with a loved one. In order to effectively solve problems, one must recognize that a problem exists, identify a desired outcome or goal that would address the problem, develop and implement a plan to obtain that goal while overcoming obstacles along the way, and evaluate the effectiveness of such a plan. When this process breaks down, be it from a skills deficit, inexperience, or avoidance and withdrawal, we become vulnerable to depression.

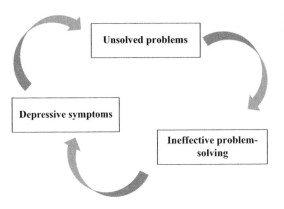

Figure 5.1 Cycle of Depression and Poor Problem-Solving

Problem-solving therapy is informed by the learned helplessness theory of depression,[3] in which individuals believe they cannot effectively solve their problems and gain control of their lives, resulting in and maintaining depression. According to PST theory, three different pathways contribute to ineffective problem-solving. First, older adults may have a *skills deficit* that is carried over from earlier learning experiences in adulthood and even childhood. Others may face new challenges because of cognitive decline, particularly in instances of executive dysfunction, which is often comorbid with late-life depression (LLD).[4] Second, even among individuals with effective problem-solving skills, some may encounter a problem with which they have *no experience* and are unable to take steps to overcome the problem. Such inexperience may be particularly relevant for older adults who are facing new demands of physical health changes, phase-of-life issues (e.g., retirement; issues of grief and loss), and other transitions associated with aging. Third, *avoidance and withdrawal* occur when individuals with otherwise effective problem-solving skills are faced with numerous or complex stressors that they cannot manage or control.

Regardless of the pathway, depression may be both a cause and an effect of decreased problem-solving ability, in which unresolved problems, resultant poor coping, low self-efficacy, and negative emotions maintain the depressive state (see Figure 5.1). Accordingly, PST aims to help individuals regain a sense of control over their problems through skills-based training which in turn, according to the theory of PST, will lead to a decrease in depressive symptomatology and improvements in functioning.

Efficacy and Effectiveness of PST

Problem-solving therapy is efficacious throughout adulthood and may be particularly relevant in addressing issues commonly faced by older adults.[5] Research has documented that skill-based psychotherapies such as PST are more effective than supportive counseling for treating LLD with comorbid medical conditions and cognitive impairment.[6,7] The structured approach of teaching straightforward, discrete steps for solving real problems is designed to address the skill deficits that can occur with disability and CI, particularly in cases of executive dysfunction. Moreover, preliminary evidence indicates that PST improves executive functioning in older adults concomitant to reduction in depression symptoms.[8]

Problem-solving therapy has also demonstrated effectiveness in treating minor depression, persistent depressive disorder (formerly dysthymia), and subsyndromal depression

(SSD).[9] This is uniquely important for older adults given the deleterious effects of even subsyndromal symptoms on health and functioning,[10] and many older adults present with clinically significant depressive symptoms that do not meet diagnostic criteria for a major depressive episode.[11] In addition to depression, PST has demonstrated preliminary evidence for treating anxiety disorders in adult primary care patients;[10] however, the literature on PST for anxiety in late life is scarce, and more research is needed to understand how to best use PST among older adults with anxiety.[12] Problem-solving therapy is not indicated as a primary treatment for substance abuse/dependence, post-traumatic stress disorder, panic disorder, new onset bipolar disorder, or new onset psychosis.

Process and Structure of Treatment

Problem-solving therapy is a short-term, goal-oriented structured psychotherapy that empowers patients to solve the "here-and-now" problems contributing to their depression. By either strengthening or reengaging their existing problem-solving abilities through direct and explicit instruction, PST teaches patients a goal-directed approach to resolving problems, resulting in greater self-efficacy and improved symptoms of depression. Such an approach requires that patients practice their skills by engaging in structured problem-solving between sessions, using a worksheet developed in session to facilitate the process. Although the main objective of this structured treatment is to teach problem-solving skills, PST is a patient-centered approach in which the clinician must maintain a collaborative therapeutic stance, develop a therapeutic alliance, and deliver treatment with empathy and support for the patient's recovery.

Problem-solving therapy typically consists of 6–12 treatment sessions which can be delivered in as little as 30 minutes per session depending on patient need and care setting. Some patients demonstrate treatment response in as few as 4 sessions, which is typically considered the minimum dose of treatment.[9] Regardless of length of treatment, PST is divided into 3 stages: (1) psychoeducation about depression and what treatment entails; (2) problem-solving skills training and active problem-solving during and between sessions; and (3) relapse prevention, which targets how to prevent relapse of a depressive episode, particularly by using the PST process for future problems.

Psychoeducation. Treatment begins with psychoeducation about depression, the link between depression and unsolved problems, and how PST fits into such a conceptualization. Many clinicians will use a weekly symptom tracker, such as the Patient Health Questionnaire (PHQ-9)[12] to assess symptoms and track treatment progress to identify when treatment intensification is necessary. During psychoeducation, the clinician can encourage collaboration by asking patients about their understanding of the depressive symptoms. In doing so, the clinician may obtain useful information about how patients appraise their current problematic situations (e.g., as challenging, unsolvable, or threatening) and their perception of their coping resources. The anticipated structure and course of PST are also discussed to acculturate the patient to this brief treatment.

Problem-Solving

The PST clinician teaches adaptive problem-solving using a seven-step approach, in which patients (1) select a specific problem and define it in concrete terms, (2) select a goal that is feasible to reach before next session, (3) brainstorm various ways to accomplish the goal, (4) evaluate the pros and cons of each solution, including the likelihood the patient can actually implement it, (5) select the best solution, (6) create a plan to implement the solution, and (7) evaluate the plan in the next session to ascertain the effectiveness of the solution.

To begin the problem-solving process, the clinician works with patients to generate a list of problems patients think are related to their depression. This can be as simple as asking, "So, what kinds of problems are you currently experiencing?" The clinician queries for *current* problems across multiple areas, including problems with family, friends, finances, occupation, health, and other social stressors (e.g., housing, transportation, legal issues). The clinician uses the comprehensive Problem List (see Figure 5.2) to facilitate this discussion. At this point, the clinician is simply noting the relevant problems that are

Problem List	
Problems with relationships (e.g., *significant other, family, friends, other*) • 18-yr-old grandson moving in • Conflict with daughter & son-in-law • Would like more friends	**Problems with daily pleasant activities:** • Given up exercise and card playing • Would like to find more social support/activities • Hasn't been reading
Problems with work or volunteer activities: • No current concerns	**Problems with sexual activity:** • No current concerns
Problems with finances: • No current concerns	**Problems with religion/spirituality/morality:** • No current concerns
Problems with housing/living arrangements: • 18-yr-old grandson moving in; need to make space • Adjustment to living with someone else • Difficulty organizing clutter	**Problems with self-image:** • Self-consciousness about exercise and card playing with increasing tremors • Would like to meet others with Parkinson's
Problems with transportation: • Takes bus–no longer drives	**Problems with aging:** • Adjustment to Parkinson's disease • Cognitive impairment – difficulty concentrating, organizing, following through on tasks
Problems with health: • Worried about Parkinson's disease • Increasing tremors • Hasn't been exercising	**Problems with loneliness:** • Social isolation, especially with worsening Parkinson's

Figure 5.2 Mrs. Rodriguez's Problem List

germane to the patient seeking treatment for depression; this is not meant to be a thorough exploration of each problem.

After generating this initial problem list, patients will select one problem to start the PST process. Rather than selecting the hardest or most daunting problem, they should be encouraged to pick a problem that they might have some ideas about already, or that they might begin addressing in the next week. Examples may include engaging in a pleasant activity, clearing clutter in the house, or strengthening a friendship. The Problem List should be referred to at each follow-up session to note progress in problem domains, add new problems, and facilitate patient selection of new problems to work on in-session.

After patients select a problem to work on in-session, clinicians orient them to the PST worksheet. This tool is jointly used in session by clinicians and patients to teach patients the seven PST steps, and then given to patients to take home as a reminder of the plan. Over the course of treatment, clinicians should facilitate patients' independence with the PST process by having patients increasingly take the initiative in creating this worksheet in session, as well as using the PST approach to solve other problems that occur between sessions. This process is illustrated in the case example below.

Case Example

Identifying information has been changed to protect the patient's privacy.

Case Introduction

Mrs. Rodriguez was a 69-year-old widowed Mexican-American woman who presented with major depressive disorder. She had a PHQ-9 score of 17, suggestive of moderately severe depressive symptomatology. Her most notable depressive symptoms were anhedonia, difficulty concentrating, difficulty with sleep onset, and feelings of worthlessness that she linked to her worsening Parkinson's disease and recent family stressors. She also had executive dysfunction secondary to Parkinson's disease, manifested behaviorally as psychomotor retardation, inertia, and difficulty planning and initiating activities. Her mental health history was negative for previous episodes of depression, although she had undergone marital counseling in her thirties. Treatment consisted of nine weekly 45-min PST sessions in a community mental health clinic.

First Session

The PST clinician began the first session with Mrs. Rodriguez by introducing herself and setting an agenda to structure the session. The clinician asked if there was anything else Mrs. Rodriguez wanted to add to the agenda to ensure a collaborative stance. In doing so, the clinician began socializing the patient to the structured and task-oriented nature of PST from the very start of their work. The session agenda consisted of the following steps:

Psychoeducation. The session began with the clinician providing an overview of the PST treatment structure. The clinician explained that each session would start with agenda setting, consisting of checking in on depressive symptoms, reviewing the action plan from the week prior, and spending the majority of the session engaging in new problem-solving, including setting an action plan for the subsequent week.

Since Mrs. Rodriguez did not have much prior experience with psychotherapy, she did not need to be resocialized to treatment as might be the case with patients who have previously participated in supportive or open-ended psychotherapies. However, the clinician still assessed Mrs. Rodriguez's expectations of psychotherapy in order to address any of her concerns. She explained how treatment would work, including the expectation that Mrs. Rodriguez would be learning and implementing a new set of skills, including between-session practice (i.e., "homework") rather than relying exclusively on discussion of her problems.

The clinician then presented the problem-solving theoretical framework and facilitated discussion of how the treatment model was relevant to the patient's life. She first explained that while everyone has problems, some individuals become overwhelmed when problems accumulate, resulting in withdrawal and feelings of hopelessness and helplessness. Mrs. Rodriguez agreed with this conceptualization and indicated that her progressing Parkinson's disease, coupled with family stressors, had left her feeling helpless and stuck. The clinician could start to use this information to leverage the introduction of the PST process: After generating a list of problems, Mrs. Rodriguez would target one problem at a time, with the intention of breaking the cycle of depression. The clinician briefly introduced the seven steps of PST. To further facilitate agreement on the use of PST strategies to treat depression, the clinician asked her to think of a time recently when she successfully solved a problem or met a goal. How did she do this? How much effort did this take? How satisfied was she with her efforts? Did she notice a boost in her mood, energy, or interest level? For instance, by discussing the challenges Mrs. Rodriguez faced in learning the bus system once she had to stop driving, and her ultimate success, the clinician reinforced this process and used it as an example for how further problem-solving efforts could proceed.

Generating the problem list. The clinician introduced the problem list and began a conversation to assess Mrs. Rodriguez's current problems (see Figure 5.2). *Note*: For clinicians in settings that do not afford a formal, standalone intake session, generating the problem list can serve a similar function to capture the most pressing problems in the "here-and-now," which is consistent with the spirit of PST and other short-term structured psychotherapies. Mrs. Rodriguez began by describing issues related to her presenting problems of Parkinson's disease and family stressors. Specifically, she noted worsening Parkinson's disease motor symptoms that had been causing her to withdraw from her previous physical activity and social activities to some degree. A key factor in her deciding to start psychotherapy, however, was the news that her 18-year-old grandson would be coming to live with her after repeated fallouts with his parents. While she was excited for the company and potential assistance, she was also nervous about the adjustment to living with someone else after being widowed for 10 years. His moving in with her was the result of his tense relationship with his parents (Mrs. Rodriguez's daughter and son-in-law), which was another source of worry and stress for Mrs. Rodriguez. She described problems concentrating on tasks that she needed to complete at home to prepare for her grandson's arrival, consistent with her executive dysfunction. The clinician then briefly probed for other domains on the problem list to obtain a thorough biopsychosocial assessment.

The clinician asked Mrs. Rodriguez to select one problem to begin working on. Although she felt pressure to prepare for her grandson's arrival, she felt a bit overwhelmed at the prospect and decided to start her first PST session by focusing on her Parkinson's disease.

Problem definition. The clinician introduced "problem definition" as the first step of PST whereby the problem is clarified and specified in concrete terms, with a particular focus on what aspects the patient may have some degree of control over. For example, clinicians may ask questions such as: What is the problem? When and where does it occur? Who is involved? How does it affect you? What have you tried to do to solve or manage it, and why are you feeling stuck now? Through this process, Mrs. Rodriguez reported that progressing Parkinson's disease was causing her frustration, particularly with regard to increased tremor activity and impaired motor ability. Clearly, the broad concept of "worsening Parkinson's disease symptoms" is a diffuse problem that is outside of anyone's control. However, PST conceptualizes problems in regard to what element of control the patient has over them – that is, defining the functional impairment and what she is doing or not doing to cope, rather than the symptom itself.

Mrs. Rodriguez was on an adequate dose of her anti-Parkinsonian medication and not yet a candidate for deep brain stimulation surgery; thus, defining the problem meant specifying exactly how her Parkinson's disease symptoms interfered with daily activities. Mrs. Rodriguez was most bothered by the withdrawal from her usual activities that she effected as a result of her worsening symptoms. She had decreased doing many of her previous activities, including physical exercise, reaching out to family and friends, and some hobbies (e.g., playing bridge). The clinician introduced the problem-solving worksheet (see Figure 5.3) and used it to coach Mrs. Rodriguez through the first step of problem definition. Through conversation, the clinician elicited details about the problem and in doing so taught Mrs. Rodriguez how to succinctly identify and define an otherwise vague, and thus unsolvable, problem.

Goal setting and generating possible solutions to reach the goal. The clinician introduced *goal setting* as something the patient would like to do differently that would be feasible to accomplish within the next week. Mrs. Rodriguez's goal was to find a suitable exercise routine that would also offer social support and interaction. The clinician guided her to select a goal that naturally followed from her problem and was clearly and succinctly defined. Mrs. Rodriguez was confident that this goal could be achieved with reasonable effort before the next session, and, thus, it did not have to be broken down into a smaller or more manageable goal.

The next step was to brainstorm a list of alternative solutions to meet her goal, a way to "wake up the brain" and counteract the depressive tendency to think that there were no good solutions, or only one "correct" option. Importantly, the clinician kept the brainstorming stage distinct from the next step in which Mrs. Rodriguez evaluated her options. This separation is important, especially early in PST, as depressed patients become accustomed to negativity bias and may automatically discount any idea they generate. By keeping the brainstorming stage separate from the evaluation stage, the clinician encouraged Mrs. Rodriguez to creatively think of a range of possible solutions and increased the chance that she would identify an effective solution. Initially, Mrs. Rodriguez had difficulty identifying more than two possible solutions; the clinician encouraged her to keep trying to come up with possibilities, with the goal of identifying at least five solutions. Rather than offering suggestions, the clinician stimulated Mrs. Rodriguez's creativity by asking her questions such as, "What else have you thought of trying?" and "What would you suggest to a friend in a similar situation?" Importantly, the clinician withheld judgment and encouraged Mrs. Rodriguez to do the same, lest a potentially successful solution be prematurely abandoned.

Evaluating and choosing the solution. Once Mrs. Rodriguez had identified five possible solutions to achieve her goal in the next week between sessions (and did not have any further ideas), the clinician guided her to strategically evaluate the alternatives by implementing

Session: **1**   Date: **Monday June 4**

1. Problem Definition: Withdrawn from exercise and social interaction since Parkinson's tremors have worsened

2. Goal: Find an exercise that is PD-friendly and would offer social support

3. Solutions:

	4. Pros	Cons
YMCA	Affordable; could try different types of exercise	Not sure if they have Parkinson's-specific activities; would have to take the bus there
Look into NW Parkinson's Foundation	Specialized resources for Parkinson's; heard good things from neurologist	Not sure what they offer
Walk with neighbor	Easy; free; neighbor is friendly	Nervous about walking difficulty; neighbor doesn't have Parkinson's
Swimming	Used to do this	Stopped doing this because of mobility difficulty and transportation
Tai Chi class	Looks relaxing & easy to do with Parkinson's	Not sure where to start looking; not sure if it would be very social

5. Choice: Look into NW Parkinson's Foundation for exercise classes/groups

6. Steps:
   a) Look at NWPF website Tuesday morning after breakfast; browse offerings
   b) Select class to attend; call to register
   c) Map out bus route
   d) Go to department store on Friday to buy new athletic outfit for class

7. Satisfaction?   ☹   ☺   ☺
                0   1   2   3   4   5   6   7   8   9   10

8. Activities for week: Go to nearby library on Wednesday; select new novel to read for at least 30 min after lunch on Wed, Sat, and Sun

Figure 5.3 Mrs. Rodriguez's Problem-Solving Worksheet

decision-making guidelines and listing pros and cons for each potential solution. The clinician then guided Mrs. Rodriguez to select a solution that was feasible, had more pros than cons identified during the evaluation process, and met her specified goal.

Implementing the preferred solution. Finally, the clinician introduced action planning as the step where Mrs. Rodriguez would create a step-by-step plan in order to execute her preferred solution before next session. For this first action plan, the clinician encouraged Mrs. Rodriguez to be particularly specific and concrete, especially given her executive dysfunction and reported difficulty concentrating and executing plans. She listed the specific steps to implement her solution (Figure 5.3). For example, she identified and listed specific sources she would contact as part of her plan. The clinician also encouraged her to identify possible obstacles. Mrs. Rodriguez noted that she might forget to start her plan. She used a pocketbook calendar to stay organized, so the clinician encouraged her to transfer some of the steps into specific days and times in the upcoming week to increase the likelihood of success. Importantly, Mrs. Rodriguez was encouraged to attempt her plan and record the outcome on her PST worksheet. The clinician reassured Mrs. Rodriguez that this next week would be an "experiment" of sorts; that is, she reassured her not to worry if the plan did not work out perfectly, as that would provide information for both of them to learn more about the problem and better understand what was going on.

Activity scheduling. Because the action plans identified in a PST session are not always immediately reinforcing or pleasant, it is important to round out a session with activity scheduling. This approach borrows from behavioral activation (BA)[13] and acknowledges that depressed individuals engage in fewer pleasurable and rewarding activities than their nondepressed counterparts, and often withdraw from and avoid such activities. Such decreased activity further maintains a person's depression. Therefore, the clinician asked Mrs. Rodriguez to identify pleasant activities she could engage in during the week and added these into her action plan. Mrs. Rodriguez suggested going to the library in her neighborhood to borrow some new books, since she had always loved reading but had not been doing much lately. She scheduled reading for 30 minutes after lunch at least three times before her next session as her pleasant activity.

Session wrap-up. The clinician summarized the session for Mrs. Rodriguez in the final minutes of their allotted session time, including the seven-step PST process. They discussed where she would keep her PST worksheet to ensure success and increase the likelihood that she would bring it to the next session for discussion. The clinician also encouraged Mrs. Rodriguez to use this framework to solve other problems before the next session.

Throughout the PST process, the clinician was empathic and took time to check in with Mrs. Rodriguez so that the approach was collaborative rather than didactic. However, the clinician did adopt an educative stance to teach Mrs. Rodriguez each step and provide a rationale for each step using easy-to-understand language in a way that engaged the patient and made sure her questions were answered.

Sessions 2–7

The second and each subsequent session began with the clinician briefly setting an agenda in order to structure the session. This included administration and review of the PHQ-9 to assess changes in depressive symptoms, review of the prior week's PST plan, review of any difficulties completing desired plans, and time dedicated to working through a new PST worksheet.

Evaluating the outcome. The seventh and final stage of PST – evaluating the outcome of the action plan from the previous session – is discussed at the start of the subsequent session. In the second session, Mrs. Rodriguez brought back her PST worksheet, allowing the clinician to review the homework with Mrs. Rodriguez and evaluate how satisfied she was with the outcome. Although she successfully identified a source for exercise by reviewing options offered by the local Parkinson's Foundation, Mrs. Rodriguez did not feel that this improved her mood over the week; indeed, her PHQ-9 score of 15 was not markedly improved. The clinician reviewed this more thoroughly, encouraging Mrs. Rodriguez to recollect her sense of satisfaction with completing her action plan and how this influenced her mood. She acknowledged that she felt a sense of accomplishment by finally making the time to find exercise options suitable to her Parkinson's disease. She also learned that the structured approach of writing out her action plan helped her feel less "scattered" than when she went about searching for activities and making phone calls to local gyms. Furthermore, she agreed that she was certainly no worse off for having started solving this problem; however, she wanted to actually start engaging in such activities, hence her lessened enthusiasm for her success. The clinician encouraged this persistence. Using a collaborative stance, the clinician and Mrs. Rodriguez agreed to continue working on this problem, with the updated goal of actually beginning her exercise routine. They worked through the remaining PST steps using the worksheet to facilitate the discussion.

At Session 3, Mrs. Rodriguez had successfully attended a local Tai Chi exercise class specifically for individuals with Parkinson's disease. She felt as though her mood improved on the days when she engaged in this activity, and she expressed hope that the class would provide not just exercise but camaraderie and social support.

At the start of Session 3, Mrs. Rodriguez also added to the agenda that she wanted to discuss her grandson's move. Since this had been a previously identified problem area, the clinician asked her how she would like to incorporate this agenda item into the session. Mrs. Rodriguez realized that she wanted some assistance working through the move, so it was incorporated into the session agenda as the focus of the PST process for the week and for a few subsequent sessions. *Note*: Some patient additions to the agenda may be simple updates that the patient wants to share with the clinician, which can therefore be incorporated into the beginning or the end of the session in a structured way that does not take time away from the PST process. Often, the addition of an agenda item may be a sign that the patient has a new, pressing problem (e.g., a conflict with a loved one, or another psychosocial issue) that may warrant the focus of the PST process.

As therapy progressed, Mrs. Rodriguez became more familiar with the steps of PST and increasingly independent in using the structured problem-solving approach, even when confronted with problems that previously left her feeling overwhelmed. As a result, she felt increasingly confident about managing and enjoying life even in the face of Parkinson's disease. She also felt increasingly at ease about her grandson coming to live with her. By Session 8, she reported that she was able to apply the problem-solving approach independently in many situations and had used the approach to find a support group for grandparents taking care of their grandchildren.

The clinician had reviewed Mrs. Rodriguez's PHQ-9 scores with her at each session, noting improvement and linking this to her effective problem-solving and persistence. At the final session, the clinician made sure to highlight Mrs. Rodriguez's markedly improved PHQ-9 score of 5 (relative to her score of 17 at Session 1) and engage her in a discussion of how the PST approach helped her manage what felt like "unsolvable" problems to feel more engaged and confident.

Relapse prevention planning. At the end of treatment, the clinician works with the patient to create a personalized relapse prevention plan, including psychoeducation on the value of relapse prevention to identify and interrupt signs of a returning depression. The clinician assists the patient in listing early warning signs of relapse, skills, and activities the patient can use to prevent depression from returning, and contact information if professional mental health care is needed in the future, while conveying optimism that the patient has the skills to address reemergence of depressive symptoms.

Special Considerations for Older Adults

As described in the case above, PST provides a particularly relevant approach to the treatment of late-life depression. It does not require any special assessment or patient selection above and beyond assessing that the patient can commit to and meaningfully engage in a brief course of psychotherapy. Problem-solving therapy directly addresses problems that are relevant and challenging for older patients by encouraging them to draw on prior experience and existing problem-solving skills while offering a concrete set of steps for approaching problems. The intervention has not been significantly modified for older adults, with the exception of taking ample time to socialize patients to the model and ensuring that the clinician appreciates the diversity of biopsychosocial problems that can arise in later life.[14]. Multiple randomized controlled trials (RCTs) have shown PST to be effective with individuals experiencing executive dysfunction,[7,15] disability,[15] acute medical issues such as stroke and cardiac disease,[16–18] and various chronic medical conditions including diabetes[19–22] and cancer.[23,24] Additional RCTs have shown PST to be effective when delivered in the home;[16,25–28] remotely via telephone or video chat;[29–31] and in various medical settings, including primary [10,24,32,33] and long-term care.[34] Problem-solving therapy has also been combined with case management to modify the intervention for older adults with significant social barriers (e.g., homebound and low-income).[7] In the next sections of the chapter, we offer a few aging-related considerations.

Mild Cognitive Impairment

Depression with cooccurring mild CI is a common presentation among older adults, particularly in the domain of executive dysfunction. Such impairment includes difficulties planning, setting goals, initiating behaviors, and organizing information, and has been shown to predict poorer treatment response in late-life depression.[7] Older adults experiencing depression and executive dysfunction typically have more difficulties completing tasks, addressing issues, and solving problems than their depressed peers without executive dysfunction.[7] Clearly, the structured approach of PST can offer a supportive framework for addressing problems despite such impairment.

Adaptations of PST for older adults with comorbid CI include having more and/or longer sessions to allow for a slower pace and better elaboration of action plans.[26] Involvement of a family member or other caregiver may be a helpful modification in this population. Such a support person can participate in most of the sessions and support problem-solving between sessions, such as assisting with the development and execution of action plans. With the patient's permission, the clinician may consider training a caregiver to be a "PST coach" for the patient, and may even provide the caregiver with an individual PST session to explain the model and its application. Such a modification can reduce depression and anxiety symptoms for a patient with CI and may serve to protect against development of depression in the caregiver.[35]

Other modifications to PST include a more active or directive stance from the clinician, including offering more direction in brainstorming efforts; encouragement to focus on less complex problems; more structure around specific steps in the action plan, goal attainment, and termination; and assistance developing cues and reminders in action plans.[7] The PST worksheet, an integral part of treatment with all populations, is particularly useful to remind patients of their plan for the week, and all patients (but particularly those with CI or other attention/concentration concerns) should be coached about where they will place the worksheet, when they will refer to it during the week, and how they may use reminders to complete the plan (e.g., setting a smartphone reminder, taping the worksheet to the bathroom mirror). Problem-solving therapy has also been modified for people with visual impairment by using tape recorders to remind patients of the PST steps and recording the outcome of action plans;[36] such approaches may also be used to support those with cognitive impairment.

Comorbid Medical Illness

Depression is common within the context of acute and chronic medical illness such as cardiovascular disease, stroke, diabetes, cancer, and arthritis, most likely due to disruptions in functional status, role, and mood, and to loss of independence.[37] The resultant disability can complicate an individual's ability to complete self-care tasks, manage health conditions, and engage in activities.

Among stroke patients, PST has been shown to delay mortality, an important finding given that poststroke depression has been associated with increased mortality even when controlling for age, physical health, and the severity of the stroke.[17,18] Treatment course can be modified such that six sessions of PST occur no later than three months poststroke coupled with six reinforcement sessions spread throughout the rest of the year.[18] Other studies have shown the efficacy of PST for older adults living with cancer,[23,24] diabetes,[19,20,22] arthritis,[38] and cardiovascular disease.[16] One RCT found that both PST and a behavioral activation treatment reduced depression and suicidal ideation (SI) in breast cancer patients.[23]

The diversity of health conditions referenced here speaks to the broad applicability of PST to older adults with both depression and chronic medical conditions, probably due to PST's focus on solving discrete problems in the here-and-now, including self-care and managing demanding treatment regimens. Across medical conditions, improved psychosocial functioning may be due in part to PST's effect on functional disability, such that improved problem-solving skills in practical domains results in improved mood and psychosocial functioning.[15]

Suicidality

Suicide rates are higher for older adults than other age cohorts, and depression is the most significant risk factor for suicidality.[39] PST, without significant modification, has been shown to be more effective than supportive therapy in reducing SI, possibly due to PST's proven effectiveness in treating depression, disability, and mild CI, three major risk factors for suicidality in older adults.[40] Given the interconnectedness of hopelessness and wishes to die, problem-solving skills may also reduce SI by generating alternatives to what may feel like unsolvable problems. For example, work by Choi and colleagues[41] offers preliminary support for the efficacy of telehealth PST in reducing SI among homebound older adults, without any specific modifications. Problem-solving therapy has also been shown to be more effective than supportive therapy in reducing SI in depressed older adults with executive dysfunction.[40]

Nontraditional Care Settings

Although many behavioral interventions have a strong evidence base for improving the symptoms of common mental health conditions, most of these were developed for specialty mental health care, with the expectation of weekly, one-hour visits from providers with extensive clinical training. Older adults may present with barriers that make it more challenging for them to receive mental health care in such traditional settings. Multiple RCTs have shown PST to be effective when delivered in primary care settings,[10,24,32,33] offered through home-based delivery,[16,25–28] and delivered remotely via telephone or video-chat.[29–31]

Primary care. One of the most effective ways to increase older adult participation in psychotherapy is by integrating such treatment into primary care, as up to 10% of older primary care patients experience clinically relevant depressive symptoms or disorders.[33] A modified version of PST for primary care (PST-PC) has been found to be effective in multiple studies. Perhaps the most widely recognized example of such integration is the IMPACT trial,[42] in which care managers were trained to deliver psychiatric services, including PST, to depressed older adults in primary care under the supervision of mental health specialists. The IMPACT project found that patients who received PST-PC had better depression outcomes, functional outcomes, and treatment adherence than those who received community-based psychotherapy.[33] Notably, PST-PC has been shown to be acceptable and effective for use by healthcare professionals without mental health experience, such as nurses.[34] PST-PC was designed to be integrated into the pace and demands of primary care settings with patients receiving between 4 and 6 sessions, with the first session lasting approximately 60 minutes and all follow-up sessions lasting no more than 30 minutes.[25,33] PST is effective in fast-paced primary care settings as it follows a brief and structured approach while remaining patient-centered and focusing on patient engagement and activation. Problem-solving therapy clinicians in such settings will likely encounter myriad issues relevant to patients in primary care, such as chronic medical disease and health promotion.

Home-based care. Older home-healthcare patients experience higher rates of depression than the general population, with some research suggesting that this group experiences depression at twice the rate of primary care patients.[16] Problem-solving therapy has been investigated in the context of home-based treatment, including the Program to Encourage Active, Rewarding Lives for Seniors (PEARLS),[43] which uses trained social service workers to deliver PST to depressed older adults in the home. Problem-solving therapy has been modified specifically for implementation in home healthcare (Brief Problem-Solving Therapy in Home Care [PST-HC][16,28]) and involves six one-hour sessions that are delivered in the patient's home by a master's level social worker. The rationale for the number of sessions, location, and choice of interventionists was driven by practicality and implementation considerations, including Medicare billing and reimbursement. Other than these structural modifications, the most notable element of PST-HC is increased flexibility in responding to the patient's medical condition, home environment, and identified needs; examples of this flexibility include different homework formats, variable session lengths, and modification of materials to meet the patient's specific presentation.[28]

Tele-health. While home healthcare is able to provide services to some older adults who are unable to access traditional mental health services, many other homebound older adults do not qualify for home health and are living in difficult-to-reach areas with limited access to formal support services. In these circumstances, utilizing telephone or video-chat technology can be useful ways to engage those individuals in mental health care. Choi et al. modified PST to be delivered via Skype (tele-PST).[29,44] Patients received six sessions of PST, with the first session taking place in person in the home to provide documents, assist with setting up the videoconferencing system, and demonstrate the use of technology; subsequent sessions were completed via Skype. Other than the delivery method, no significant modifications to the PST structure were made.[29,45] This study found tele-PST to be as effective as in-person PST offered in the patient's home in reducing depression and disability, and showed high levels of acceptance of tele-PST in this population.[29]

Cultural Modifications and Other Considerations

Problem-solving therapy has also been modified to respond to a variety of cultural considerations. Notably, PST has been translated into multiple languages, including Spanish, Hebrew, French, and Chinese; translated materials are available through the National Network of PST Clinicians, Trainers, and Researchers (https://pstnetwork.ucsf .edu/; Director: P. Raue). While language translation is of obvious importance, it is equally important to consider modifications to the delivery of PST within specific cultural groups. One example of this being done is a modification to PST known as Problem-Solving Therapy–Chinese Older Adult (PST-COA),[46] which maintains the primary structure of PST while incorporating modifications specific to this population, including having the clinician provide more suggestions during the brainstorming phase to maintain the clinician's position as an authority figure.[46] In PST-COA and all iterations of PST, it is the clinician's responsibility to ensure that the material, structure, and topics are presented in a culturally responsive manner that meets the needs and expectations of the patient.

Despite the structure of PST, clinicians should retain a patient-centered approach in treatment. Clinicians should consider cultural factors, previous exposure to psychotherapy, biopsychosocial stressors, and socioeconomic background, and how such factors may influence the patient's acceptance of and engagement with PST. For example, although older adults are generally receptive to the goal-directed approach, some individuals may initially find PST to be too formal or mechanical, as with any brief behavioral treatment. While the structured nature of PST can be a powerful tool with which individuals can make progress in a short course of therapy, it is important that clinicians respond appropriately to the patient's unique biopsychosocial presentation. Clinicians should consider modifications that stick to the spirit of PST when such structure or forms are not well received; examples include deploying the seven steps of PST in a more conversational fashion, relying less on formal worksheets, and allowing protected time for general "check-ins" about factors affecting the patient that are not the focus of the problem-solving process. The elements of PST that make it effective include patient understanding and acceptance of PST's action-oriented framework, patient engagement in action planning and implementation, and the clinician using compassionate time management and thoughtful redirection in order to maintain the structure and spirit of PST within sessions. Finally, as with all treatment approaches, the clinician should consider how well PST is working for the individual patient at hand, based on measurement-based care and patient reports of progress and intervention fit.

Training and Other PST Resources

If readers would like to pursue training and certification in PST, we encourage them to visit the University of Washington's AIMS (Advancing Integrated Mental Health Solutions) Center website on Behavioral Interventions at https://aims.uw.edu/collaborative-care/behav ioral-interventions, and to contact uwaims@uw.edu.

Conclusion

Problem-solving therapy's demonstrated effectiveness in treating LLD across practice settings and patient populations presents clinicians with a treatment option that is both effective and accessible. The present-orientation and problem-solving focus of PST allows for clinicians and patients to address issues that impact the patient's current quality of life, health, and overall wellbeing. Problem-solving therapy may be particularly relevant for offsetting skill deficits associated with LLD in instances of mild CI (especially executive dysfunction) and disability. Emerging research into the implementation of PST continues to consider contextual factors to improve treatment delivery. Priority should be given to recruiting and training the geriatric mental health workforce to deliver evidence-based psychosocial interventions in older adults, including PST.

References

1. D'Zurilla TJ. *Problem-solving therapy: a social competence approach to clinical intervention.* New York: Springer; 1986.

2. Nezu CM, Perri MG, Nezu AM. *Problem-solving therapy for depression: theory, research, and clinical guidelines.* New York: Wiley; 1989.

3. Seligman ME. *Depression and learned helplessness. The psychology of depression: contemporary theory and research.* Oxford: John Wiley & Sons; 1974. p. xvii, 318.

4. Alexopoulos GS, Kiosses DN, Klimstra S, Kalayam B, Bruce ML. Clinical presentation of the "depression–executive dysfunction syndrome" of late life. *Am J Geriatr Psychiatry.* 2002;10(1):98–106.

5. Kiosses DN, Alexopoulos GS. Problem-solving therapy in the elderly. *Curr Treat Options Psych.* 2014;1(1):15–26.

6. Cuijpers P, Karyotaki E, Pot AM, Park M, Reynolds CF. Managing depression in older age: psychological interventions. *Maturitas.* 2014;79(2):160–169.

7. Areán PA, Raue P, Mackin RS, et al. Problem-solving therapy and supportive therapy in older adults with major depression and executive dysfunction. *Am J Psychiatry.* 2010;167(11):1391–1398.

8. Mackin RS, Nelson JC, Delucchi K, et al. Cognitive outcomes after psychotherapeutic interventions for major depression in older adults with executive dysfunction. *Am J Geriatr Psychiatry.* 2014;22(12):1496–1503.

9. Williams JJW, Barrett J, Oxman T, et al. Treatment of dysthymia and minor depression in primary care: a randomized controlled trial in older adults. *JAMA.* 2000;284(12):1519–1526.

10. Zhang AA, Park S, Sullivan J, Jing SJ. The effectiveness of problem-solving therapy for primary care patients' depressive and/or anxiety disorders: a systematic review and meta-analysis. *J Am Board Fam Med.* 2018; 31:139–150.

11. Kasckow JW, Karp JF, Whyte E, et al. Subsyndromal depression and anxiety in older adults: health related, functional, cognitive and diagnostic implications. *J Psychiatr Res.* 2013;47(5):599–603.

12. Kroenke K, Spitzer RL, Williams JBW. The PHQ-9 validity of a brief depression severity measure. *J Gen Intern Med.* 2001;16(9):606–613.

13. Lejuez CW, Hopko DR, Acierno R, Daughters SB, Pagoto SL. Ten year revision of the brief behavioral activation treatment for depression: revised treatment manual. *Behav Modif.* 2011;35 (2):111–161.

14. Crabb RC, Areán PA. Problem-solving treatment for late-life depression. In: Areán, PA, editor. *Treatment of late-life depression, anxiety, trauma, and substance abuse.* Washington, DC: American Psychological Association; 2015.

15. Alexopoulos GS, Raue PJ, Kiosses DN, et al. Problem-solving therapy and supportive therapy in older adults with major depression and executive dysfunction:

effect on disability. *Arch Gen Psychiatry.* 2011;**68**(1):33–41.

16. Gellis ZD, Bruce ML. Problem-solving therapy for subthreshold depression in home healthcare patients with cardiovascular disease. *Am J Geriatr Psychiatry.* 2010;**18**(6):464–474.

17. Robinson RG, Jorge RE, Long J. Prevention of poststroke mortality using problem-solving therapy or escitalopram. *Am J Geriatr Psychiatry.* 2017;**25**(5):512–519.

18. Robinson RG, Jorge RE, Moser DJ, et al. Escitalopram and problem-solving therapy for prevention of poststroke depression: a randomized controlled trial. *JAMA.* 2008;**299**(20):2391–2400.

19. Villamil-Salcedo V, Vargas-Terrez BE, Caraveo-Anduaga J, et al. Glucose and cholesterol stabilization in patients with type 2 diabetes mellitus with depressive and anxiety symptoms by problem-solving therapy in primary care centers in Mexico City. *Prim Health Care Res Dev.* 2018;**19**(1):33–41.

20. Hoseini Z, Azkhosh M, Younesi J, Soltani E. The effectiveness of problem solving therapy on coping skills in women with type 2 diabetes. *Iranian Rehabilitation Journal.* 2014;**12**(2):39–43.

21. Taveira TH, Dooley AG, Cohen LB, Khatana SAM, Wu W-C. Pharmacist-led group medical appointments for the management of type 2 diabetes with comorbid depression in older adults. *Ann Pharmacother.* 2011;**45**(11):1346–1355.

22. Katon W, Unützer J, Fan M-Y, et al. Cost-effectiveness and net benefit of enhanced treatment of depression for older adults with diabetes and depression. *Diabetes Care.* 2006;**29**(2):265.

23. Hopko DR, Funderburk JS, Shorey RC, et al. Behavioral activation and problem-solving therapy for depressed breast cancer patients: preliminary support for decreased suicidal ideation. *Behav Modif.* 2013;**37**(6):747–767.

24. Fann JR, Fan M-Y, Unützer J. Improving primary care for older adults with cancer and depression. *J Gen Intern Med.* 2009;**24**(2):417–424.

25. Choi NG, Marti CN, Bruce ML, Hegel MT. Depression in homebound older adults: problem-solving therapy and personal and social resourcefulness. *Behav Ther.* 2013;**44**(3):489–500.

26. Kiosses DN, Teri L, Velligan DI, Alexopoulos GS. A home-delivered intervention for depressed, cognitively impaired, disabled elders. *Int J Geriatr Psychiatry.* 2011;**26**(3):256–262.

27. Kiosses DN, Areán PA, Teri L, Alexopoulos GS. Home-delivered problem adaptation therapy (PATH) for depressed, cognitively impaired, disabled elders: a preliminary study. *Am J Geriatr Psychiatry.* 2010;**18**(11):988–998.

28. Gellis Z, McGinty J, Horowitz A, Bruce M, Misener E. Problem-solving therapy for late-life depression in home care: a randomized field trial. *Am J Geriatr Psychiatry.* 2007;**15**(11):968–978.

29. Choi NG, Marti CN, Marinucci ML, et al. Telehealth problem-solving therapy for depressed low-income homebound older adults. *Am J Geriatr Psychiatry.* 2013;**22**(3).

30. Arnaert A, Klooster J, Chow V. Attitudes towards videotelephones: an exploratory study of older adults with depression. *J Gerontol Nurs.* 2007;**33**(9):5–13.

31. Kleiboer A, Donker T, Seekles W, et al. A randomized controlled trial on the role of support in internet-based problem solving therapy for depression and anxiety. *Behav Res Ther.* 2015;**72**:63–71.

32. Nguyen CM, Chen KH, Denburg NL. The use of problem-solving therapy for primary care to enhance complex decision-making in healthy community-dwelling older adults. *Front Psychol.* 2018;**9**:870.

33. Areán P, Hegel M, Vannoy S, Fan M-Y, Unützer J. Effectiveness of problem-solving therapy for older, primary care patients with depression: results from the IMPACT project. *The Gerontologist.* 2008;**48**(3):311–323.

34. Reinhardt JP, Horowitz A, Cimarolli VR, Eimicke JP, Teresi JA. Addressing depression in a long-term care setting: a phase II pilot of problem-solving

treatment. *Clin Ther.* 2014;**36** (11):1531–1537.

35. Stahl ST, Rodakowski J, Gildengers AG, et al. Treatment considerations for depression research in older married couples: a dyadic case study. *Am J Geriatr Psychiatry.* 2017;**25**(4):388–395.

36. Rovner BW, Casten RJ, Hegel MT, Leiby BE, Tasman WS. Preventing depression in age-related macular degeneration. *Arch Gen Psychiatry.* 2007;**64**(8):886–892.

37. Raue P, McGovern A, Kiosses D, Sirey J. Advances in psychotherapy for depressed older adults. *Cur Psychiatry Rep.* 2017;**19** (9):1–9.

38. Lin EHB, Katon W, Von Korff M, et al. Effect of improving depression care on pain and functional outcomes among older adults with arthritis: a randomized controlled trial. *JAMA.* 2003;**290** (18):2428–2429.

39. Fiske A, Wetherell JL, Gatz M. Depression in older adults. *Annu Rev Clin Psychol.* 2009;5:363–389.

40. Gustavson KA, Alexopoulos GS, Niu GC, et al. Problem-solving therapy reduces suicidal ideation in depressed older adults with executive dysfunction. *Am J Geriatr Psychiatry.* 2016;**24**(1):11–7.

41. Choi NG, Marti CN, Conwell Y. Effect of problem-solving therapy on depressed low-income homebound older adults' death/suicidal ideation and hopelessness. *Suicide Life Threat Behav.* 2016;**46** (3):323–336.

42. Unützer J, Katon W, Callahan CM, et al. Collaborative care management of late-life depression in the primary care setting: a randomized controlled trial. *JAMA.* 2002;**288**(22):2836–2845.

43. Ciechanowski P, Wagner E, Schmaling K, et al. Community-integrated home-based depression treatment in older adults: a randomized controlled trial. *JAMA.* 2004;**291**(13):1569–1577.

44. Choi NG, Sirey JA, Bruce ML. Depression in homebound older adults: recent advances in screening and psychosocial interventions. *Curr Transl Geriatr Exp Gerontol Rep.* 2013;2(1):16.

45. Choi NG, Hegel MT, Sirrianni L, Marinucci ML, Bruce ML. Passive coping response to depressive symptoms among low-income homebound older adults: Does it affect depression severity and treatment outcome? *Behav Res Ther.* 2012;**50** (11):668–674.

46. Chu JP, Huynh L, Areán P. Cultural adaptation of evidence-based practice utilizing an iterative stakeholder process and theoretical framework: problem solving therapy for Chinese older adults. *Int J Geriatr Psychiatry.* 2012;27(1): 97–106.

Chapter

Interpersonal Psychotherapy in Later Life

Mark D. Miller and Richard K. Morycz

Introduction, Overview, and Basics

Interpersonal psychotherapy (IPT) is a short-term, evidenced-based treatment, originally developed as a therapy for depression. It has been subsequently adapted for various subgroups including geriatric patients. Interpersonal psychotherapy is empirically derived with contributions from Harry Stack Sullivan and Adolf Meyer, who recognized that the role of the patient's psychosocial setting and interpersonal experience had a profound effect on symptom development.

Three component processes in IPT are defined as:

1. *Symptom Formation*, which refers to depressed affect and neurovegetative symptoms of depression.
2. *Social and interpersonal relations* and interactions with others in one or more social roles. These forces are shaped by childhood learning, personal experiences to date, and current social reinforcement. This component led to the concept of four main foci of IPT (role transition, unresolved grief, role dispute, and interpersonal deficit). Intervention in IPT thus focuses on social roles and interpersonal relationships, and asks what changes could be achieved for patients in order to improve their particular situations in such a way as to decrease depressive symptoms and improve function.
3. *Personality factors* are seen as enduring traits that are essentially fixed early in life and are not easily modified, especially in a short-term treatment. Various maladaptive coping styles frequently seen in those with personality disorders can affect self-esteem, communications styles, interpersonal sensitivity, and expressions of anger and guilt. Personality factors are recognized as a potential contributing factor to the onset or maintenance of depressive symptoms but are not a focus of treatment in IPT. It is further recognized that successful symptom reduction and improved social functioning can reduce the intensity of personality traits.[1]

Another contribution to the development of IPT is based on attachment theory, in which John Bowlby emphasized how early-life attachments can profoundly impact feelings of security, which, in turn, form the basis for the quality of all subsequent relationships. The ability to develop deep affectional bonds with primary support figures impacts growing children's comfort levels in exploring their world and making attachments in other social groups. While IPT recognizes the early-life antecedents of personality development, in contrast to psychoanalysis, which focuses heavily on these forces, IPT merely focuses on the extent to which those forces are playing out in *present* relationships and asks the question: Despite past formative forces that cannot be undone, what strategies can patients use to acknowledge the proximal contribution of these developmental forces in their current depressive symptoms, and what changes can be implemented to improve current interpersonal relationships and therefore reduce depressive symptoms?[2]

For patients suffering from depression with low energy, low motivation, and poor concentration, being less efficient or unable to perform in their usual capacity is common. The IPT therapist thus gives patients permission to allow themselves to temporarily assume the *sick role* in a similar way that being physically ill from pneumonia would preclude carrying out their usual duties until the symptoms of illness improved and patients began to feel more like their old selves again. In concrete terms, if one were diagnosed with pneumonia, raking leaves would not be expected but rather bed rest, chicken soup, and possibly taking antibiotics until the infection clears and strength returns to normal. The IPT therapist points out that severe depression can also be debilitating even if it is not as visually obvious.

The biological or genetic underpinnings of depression are advancing rapidly with new technologies for probing the brain. These forces are also recognized in IPT, and the concomitant use of pharmacologic or somatic treatments is accepted as another evidence-based treatment approach. An IPT therapist supports compliance with medication in those patients receiving combination treatment, and this psychoeducational effort may improve outcomes for those patients who require such treatment.

In summary, IPT focuses on interpersonal and social functioning or events in the recent past that appear to have triggered or contributed to depressive symptoms. Interpersonal psychotherapy recognizes the contribution of early life events, personality traits, and biological or genetic contributions to the onset and maintenance of depression but does not focus on them.

Focus Areas

Interpersonal psychotherapy specifically concentrates on four areas of focus: role transitions, unresolved grief, role disputes, and interpersonal deficits. These categories are not mutually exclusive; however, a main focus is usually identified.

1. *Role transitions* can include changes in major life events (such as divorce, changes in living arrangements, retirement, raising grandchildren, recent changes in functioning due to acute or chronic medical problems, or even self-awareness of changes in cognitive capabilities).
2. *Unresolved grief* follows the death of someone who is important in the life of the patient.
3. *Role disputes* can be recent or long-standing interpersonal conflicts typically involving a partner or spouse, an adult child, a parent, or a close friend. In later life, role disputes can result when adult children move back into the homes of their parents for economic reasons or when they volunteer or become tasked with raising grandchildren when their own children become ill, die, struggle with substance abuse, or become incarcerated.
4. Finally, *interpersonal deficits* can lead to distress or depression from maladaptive personality traits that are intensified by stress or changing circumstances. Goals and interventions of IPT are rooted in real life and the current reality and circumstances of the patient. Prior traumatic or early life events are acknowledged but not a focus of treatment.

The Structure of IPT

Interpersonal psychotherapy is divided into three simple phases:

1. Early sessions (2–3)
2. Middle sessions (8–12)
3. Termination sessions (2–3)

After a patient with significant symptoms of depression is properly evaluated, including the diagnosis and treatment of any medical conditions that might be contributing to depression, such as hypothyroidism or vitamin B12 deficiency, the patient is assessed for the appropriateness of somatic treatment, psychotherapy, or their combination. Patient preference is also taken into account. For any psychotherapy to be successful, a good working rapport is required to educate the patient about depression and to build a mutually trusting and safe environment for the work of psychotherapy to begin. If IPT is chosen as the psychotherapy to be applied, the IPT therapist uses the information gathered to formulate a proposed plan for the therapeutic work ahead. The IPT therapist chooses the most appropriate of the four foci that will guide the therapy along a set of predetermined guidelines, and this plan is presented to the patient for consideration in the context of the solicited clinical history. If this interpretation of the linkages between the onset of the most recent depressive symptoms or declining function is acceptable to the patient, a therapeutic contract is established with an agreement to meet weekly for 12–16 face-to-face sessions and be psychologically open to understanding the underpinnings of the event(s) or circumstances that immediately preceded the onset of depressive symptoms with particular attention paid to changes in social roles that led to demoralization and depression. This agreement or treatment contract will become important later in the intermediate phase of treatment to remind the patient that limited time remains to complete the work before termination in the agreed timeframe (conscious and unconscious pressure), and thus working hard toward agreed upon goals is strongly encouraged. A useful construct for some IPT therapists is the creation of an "illness timeline" to search for links to the onset of depressive symptoms in the context of well-known time points such as national holidays or birthdays.

Early Sessions

During the first two to three sessions, the IPT therapist identifies the focus or problem area based on all information gathered to that point, presents a contract for 12–16 weekly sessions to focus on the problem area that has been agreed to by the patient (and caregiver(s) in IPT for cognitive impairment [IPT-ci]), and assigns the patient the "sick role." Next on the agenda is the *interpersonal inventory* of all significant family members and other important relationships. The IPT therapist begins with the persons with whom the patient lives, an inventory of all family members, noting something about the quality of that relationship in modest but not exhaustive detail (including those who have recently died). Is it a good relationship, a supportive one, or is it burdensome or contentious, distant or neglectful? This exercise can identify current and potential supports who could be potentially reactivated by the patient to improve social interaction. The interpersonal inventory will also discover problematic relationships that are potential or current role disputes. Some IPT therapists prefer to draw a traditional family tree and also identify any significant nonfamily members important to the patient, such as friends, supportive clergy, romantic interests, or contentious relationships with employers or neighbors, and so on. Recently deceased individuals of importance are also included. For a therapy based on interpersonal relations, the interpersonal inventory comprises the individuals in the patient's sphere of interaction where the work of IPT is carried out. The key is to identify those relationships that may, through absence or conflict, relate to the patient's current depression or lost function. Useful lines of questioning to complete the goals for the interpersonal inventory include exploring what kinds of relationships are available, their quality (confidant?), frequency of contact, availability, and degree of reciprocity.

The IPT therapist plays an active role as an advocate and facilitator who helps the patient to brainstorm about options for alternative coping strategies, encourages improved social interactions, and ultimately fosters competence to do the same on the patient's own recognizance within 12–16 weeks when termination is completed. There is activity and engagement on the part of the therapist (including direct suggestions). To borrow from psychodynamic terminology, a strong therapeutic alliance is important. Identifying and concentrating on a problem area is essential. The IPT approach utilizes the medical model of illness for depression. The therapist's task is for the patient to understand linkages between mood and life events, activities, and relationships. During treatment sessions, the therapist is a supportive coach, ally, teacher, and reinforcer. Besides the social support network scan, early sessions of therapy are focused upon the therapeutic alliance, diagnosing depression, having the patient accept the medical model of depression and the sick role, identifying and establishing the problem area with the patient, providing psychoeducation, and fostering hope.

Middle Sessions

Interpersonal psychotherapy in the middle sessions of treatment utilizes specific objectives and interventions related to each problem area that is outlined in manual form, with specific, detailed approaches for each of the four problem areas or foci (role dispute, unresolved grief, role transition, and interpersonal deficit).

The IPT therapist specifically encounters and responds to patients' needs, abilities, wishes, plans, and emotional expressions through brainstorming sessions where patients are asked to think of and consider alternate coping strategies that might work better to meet their goals. Every effort is made to encourage patients to do the "work" of the exploration. Termination is constantly on the mind of the IPT therapist, where patients will soon be expected to carry out the same exercise on their own. The IPT therapist facilitates the brainstorming sessions but only offers direct suggestions when the patient appears to be stuck, thus avoiding undue dependence on the therapist to give advice or solve problems. Patients who are struggling with difficult issues and are able to generate their own possible alternative strategies and resolve to try their implementation of the new strategies will gain more of a sense of ownership and mastery, particularly if the linkage between successful implementation and the drop in their depression severity score is repeatedly pointed out to them. Patients are encouraged to take action, to take risks in real-life social interactions and meaningful activities.

Termination Sessions

During the last several sessions, the therapist discusses termination, and promotes and summarizes the patient's capabilities and achievements during treatment. Within the IPT process, patients may succeed in modifying interpersonal encounters and tasks, or they may fall short in reaching problem-area objectives in any given week. If positive interpersonal goals are achieved, the therapist maintains a supportive stance, reinforces the success, and clarifies the interpersonal skills that were utilized. When attempts to achieve goals are disappointing, the therapist is still supportive, shows understanding and sympathy, evaluates what went awry, and assists in more brainstorming to try another approach. Hope is promoted, and reassurance is provided. The beginning of each session should include a review of events since the last session and a reporting of the successes and challenges of interpersonal strategies attempted in the patient's life. At the end of each session, new strategies and accomplishments are summarized.

IPT and Older Persons

Interpersonal psychotherapy is especially suited for use with older persons, as they are at risk for social isolation within the context of depression when relationships are changed, disrupted, in conflict, or gone. Social isolation puts them at even more risk for premature mortality and for morbidity. Interpersonal therapy can help promote social ties and supports.

Interpersonal psychotherapy is a practical psychotherapy for use with older patients for the following reasons. Interpersonal psychotherapy seems to the patient like a conversation with a concerned provider and does not involve terms to learn, homework, or jargon. Interpersonal psychotherapy allows patients to "tell their story" of current difficulties and then focuses more narrowly to intervene. Interpersonal psychotherapy is straightforward in its approach by focusing only on the here-and-now not the distant past, which is useful for teaching beginning therapists. Interpersonal psychotherapy can be taught to social workers and nurses as well as psychologists and physicians. The PROSPECT[3] and IMPACT[4] studies taught us that having a mental health professional for regular consultation or a mental health provider imbedded within a primary care practice can hasten the resolution of depression and suicidal ideation (SI) as well as promote the acceptance of psychotherapy in patients who would otherwise not seek it. Three of the four main foci of IPT (unresolved grief, role transition, and role dispute) are common causes of distress, depression, or anxiety in older patients

Interpersonal psychotherapy is a time-limited but powerful psychotherapy for focusing on one or two problem areas, which is attractive for older patients who are worried about long-term commitments and/or the cost of long-term therapy.

Coping with increasing disability among older patients is mitigated by a robust support system, which IPT encourages and seeks to repair when broken. Interpersonal psychotherapy offers a monthly maintenance version, particularly for those with a history of chronic role disputes, in order to maintain gains achieved through more adaptive coping strategies provided in the acute phase of IPT. Interpersonal psychotherapy is also fully compatible with the use of psychotropic medication that can be managed in a single follow-up session with a provider with prescribing privileges or in a primary care office with an IPT therapist onsite.

By engaging concerned accompanying caregivers from the outset, utilizing a combination of individual or joint sessions as indicated, and seeking a steady state of compensated functionality with varying follow-up intervals as needed for the remaining life of the patient, IPT and its derivative IPT-ci for cognitively impaired patients and caregivers allows for seamless treatment of older patients who present with major depression, CI, or their combination.

Interpersonal psychotherapy focuses on relationships, particularly when connectedness to others is strained, broken, damaged, or missing, secondary to depression or CI in later life. Affected individuals can lose a sense of relatedness and become isolated. Interpersonal psychotherapy treatment techniques thus explore the intimate and meaningful aspects of persons' lives, as strong therapeutic relationships can promote, restore, and enhance the wellbeing of individuals and buffer stress. Interpersonal psychotherapy seeks to improve relationships and social connectedness to reduce depressive symptoms and improve overall function.

Practical Issues of Implementing IPT with Elders

No major adaptation of IPT is required for use with older patients. It is highly recommended to have a working knowledge of the basics of gerontology to be familiar with common problems facing elders. Hearing loss may impair good communication, and therefore positioning one's chair on the side of the patient's "best ear" in closer proximity may help.[5] Transportation can be problematic, especially in inclement weather, during which telephone visits can be substituted, or entire courses of IPT can be carried out by telephone if the patient has adequate privacy and can hear well enough. Caregivers may accompany older patients and want to sit in or receive progress reports, which must be negotiated with the patient. Although there is a couples therapy version of IPT, it was designed as an individual psychotherapy. For an elderly person who comes with a selfless and supportive caregiver, the identified patient still deserves the right to privacy for individual therapy and may need to complain about a well-meaning caregiver as overbearing or stifling. Those patients who present with significant CI may be best served by implementing IPT-ci, in which caregivers are incorporated into the treatment from the beginning, thus avoiding the perception of a change in therapeutic technique later in treatment when it may prove necessary for the patient's safety or welfare. In IPT-ci, the therapist exercises discretion about a combination of individual sessions with the identified patient or family member or caregiver, or joint sessions, as appropriate. For older patients who may suffer from chronic pain or other discomforts, some flexibility in the length of sessions may be necessary from 40-60 minutes.

Involving Caregivers When Cognitive Impairment Is Involved

In the assessment and treatment of older individuals where CI is part of the clinical picture, the IPT therapist considers using principles of IPT for cognitive impairment. The techniques of IPT-ci are designed to involve caregivers from the outset of treatment by soliciting their ongoing input and utilizing their skills and availability for the benefit of identified patients. These techniques are particularly important if patients show signs of executive dysfunction, which are often misrecognized or poorly understood by family members or caregivers as being unwanted behaviors that are perceived to be deliberate, hurtful, or just uncaring. For patients who have little insight into the nature of their problematic or maladaptive behaviors due to CI, an alliance with one or more caregivers can soften any negative consequences and improve tolerance and respect for patients who are not aware of how they are perceived by others. The IPT-ci therapist is an advocate for identified patients and caregivers insofar as caregivers need understanding and support for optimizing their caregiver skills. Caregivers may need their own support for other problem areas in their lives (such as problems with their own children, spouses, or workplace stresses). The IPT therapist also realizes that caregivers are often going through their own role transition from adult child to caregiver, which might generate role disputes with their parents. Caregivers may also need legal advice for wills or medical power-of-attorney documents, advanced directives, and social services for finding paid help, alternate housing, and perhaps a nursing home or long-term care facility. For the unseasoned IPT-ci therapist, the collective problems of the identified patient plus the caregiver can seem daunting or confusing, which is why it is necessary to clearly define the role of the IPT-ci therapist as an advocate for the patient. In rare circumstances, elder abuse may be taking place (financial, emotional, physical, sexual abuse, or neglect) such that IPT therapists are obligated to report this abuse to the appropriate authority as they would in any case of child abuse.

The Efficacy of IPT in Late Life

Both IPT and antidepressant medications have been independently shown to significantly reduce depressive symptoms more than placebo or waitlist controls in adults.[6]

Interpersonal psychotherapy has been shown to be by itself an efficacious and user-friendly treatment for depression in later life or as an adjunct to or in combination with antidepressant medication.[7] Most studies focus on the combined use of medication and IPT, however, thus making it more difficult to discern the effects of IPT directly.

In a group of 143 depressed elders seen in a primary care setting in the Netherlands, IPT showed superior efficacy to treatment as usual (TAU).[8] Post et al. further review the use of IPT in older primary care patients.[9]

Given that unresolved grief is one of the four foci of IPT, and losses through death are more common in late life, Miller describes applying IPT to spousal bereavement.[10] However, a randomized controlled trial of IPT, nortriptyline, and their combination compared to clinical management (CM) for bereavement-related depression in elders did not show a benefit for IPT over CM, or an added benefit for IPT to nortriptyline alone. Those assigned to IPT, however, did show fewer dropouts compared to clinical management.[11]

In a series of studies patterned after the classic collaborative study of maintenance therapy in adults,[12] Reynolds et al. completed three acute and maintenance studies of late-life depression. The first used combined treatment with antidepressant medication plus IPT for up to 26 weeks to achieve full remission, defined as a Hamilton Rating Scale for Depression (HAM-D) score of 10 or less. Remitters were randomized to a combination of drug plus IPT, drug plus CM, pill placebo plus IPT, or pill placebo plus clinical management. In the Maintenance Therapies in Late-Life Depression (MTLD) study, the drug was nortriptyline, age was restricted to between 60 and 79, all subjects were required to be cognitively intact by a screening test cut-off score, and all had to have at least one prior lifetime episode of major depression (i.e., recurrent depression). Remitters were followed with monthly visits for three years. Results showed that all three active treatment cells were statistically superior to the pill-placebo-plus-CM group, which showed an 80% recurrence rate. The group with the lowest recurrence rate (20%) was the combination drug-plus-IPT group, with reduced efficacy for drug-plus-CM and pill-placebo-plus-IPT, respectively, although all were statistically superior to pill-placebo-plus-clinical-management. In this group of elders with recurrent depression, the pill-placebo-plus-IPT group was also superior to pill-placebo-plus-CM, indicating a protective effect of IPT alone on recurrences of major depression.[13]

Interestingly, in this last subgroup a closer look at the data of the placebo-plus-IPT compared to the placebo-plus-CM group revealed a statistically higher recurrence rate in subjects with an IPT problem area of role dispute during the acute phase of combined therapy if they were subsequently randomly assigned to CM in maintenance versus monthly IPT refresher sessions. This suggests a need for continued monthly IPT sessions to maintain psychotherapeutic gains achieved in the acute phase of treatment with an original IPT focus of role dispute.[14] No statistical difference prevailed among the other IPT foci, suggesting that a grief or role transition focus may have been adequately resolved in the acute phase of treatment, whereas the gains made in finding new strategies for coping better with chronic role disputes in the acute phase may have dwindled over time in the CM group, leading to demoralization and an eventual recurrence of major depression compared to those assigned to monthly IPT sessions where those gains or new coping strategies were maintained.

In the MTLD-II study, older adults aged 70 years and older were treated similarly with combined antidepressant drug paroxetine and IPT, although there was no requirement for a prior recurrent depression history. Remitters were randomized for follow-up. In this study, there was no added protective benefit of IPT to drug alone in rates of protection against a recurrence.[15] Compared to the original MTLD cohort, this group was 10 years older and had significantly more medical burden, suggesting that the strength of the drug effect required to achieve remission may have overshadowed any contribution from IPT. This sample also differed in that subjects with mild CI were not excluded as in the original study. The IPT group did show a longer time to recurrence compared to the CM group among the subset who showed mild cognitive impairment.[16]

In the third and final MTLD study, escitalopram was used as the antidepressant drug in a sample of 128 elders with major depression in which both the IPT and CM group showed efficacy in preventing recurrences when combined with the drug but no statistical added benefit for IPT over clinical management.[17] Arean and Cook offer a concise comparative review of various psychotherapies alone or in combination with pharmacotherapy.[18]

Taken together these studies suggest that IPT is acceptable and efficacious in treating late-life depression to remission, particularly when combined with antidepressant medication. For elders with more accumulated medical problems or chronic pain or higher initial severity of depression, antidepressant medication appears to be required to maintain remission.[19] Although there was no added benefit for IPT over CM, the reader should bear in mind that CM is not a "no treatment" condition but a form of supportive therapy that provides psychoeducation about the risks and underpinnings of depressive symptoms, the rationale for treatment, and the specific challenges to resistance to stay in treatment. In other words, in the real world of TAU, a difference between IPT and TAU may have been detectable, since IPT provides all the benefits of TAU plus other specific psychotherapeutic interventions within the four focus areas of role transition, grief, role dispute, and interpersonal deficit.

Given the common presentation of older patients with depression combined with CI, an adaptation of IPT was developed by Miller et al.[20,21] to acknowledge the important and sometimes complex roles the caregiver plays in the treatment of depression, as well as in the concomitant management of cognitive impairment. This adaptation was published in manual form.[22] A small unpublished trial of IPT-ci was undertaken after it was taught to nurse-practitioners and social workers, who applied its principles to consecutive patients enrolled in a multidisciplinary geriatric treatment center (Benedum Geriatric Center in Pittsburgh) after institutional review board (IRB) approval and patient and caregiver consent were obtained. The IPT-ci techniques were broadly accepted by both patients and caregivers. An unpublished analysis of the first 15 patients showed that scores on the Montreal Cognitive Assessment (MoCA)[23] ranged from 12–28 and on the PHQ-9 from 3–22 at baseline.[24] Thirteen patients were accompanied by caregivers, six of whom were spouses and the remainder adult children. The established IPT focus area was role transition to a less functional state in 14 patients and interpersonal deficit in one case. Ten subjects showed a baseline of 10 or higher on the PHQ-9 scores with a mean of 17.6 at baseline, 10.2 at three months, 9.1 at six months, and 7.5 at 12 months. Nonparametric statistical comparisons of change from baseline to three months were: n = 9, p = 0.0625; to six months, n = 9, p = 0.0078; and to 12 months, n = 7, p = 0.0313. Repeat MoCA scores at 12 months did not change or trended lower. No changes in antidepressant medications were made during the follow-up period. This open trial demonstrated the acceptability and feasibility of delivering IPT-ci in a real-world setting, and these preliminary results demonstrated a downward trend in depression severity over time. Further research is needed to validate these results.

In conclusion, the evidence base shows that IPT appears to be a robust treatment for mild to moderate depression alone, a powerful treatment in combination with antidepressants for acute treatment, an effective monthly maintenance treatment against recurrence in the "young old" (aged 60–70 years), with a particular benefit for those with an IPT focus in the acute phase on role dispute. In older individuals with depression and concomitant mild-to-moderate cognitive dysfunction, an adaptation of IPT called IPT-ci (for cognitive impairment) includes caregivers as an integral part of the treatment and showed a reduction of depression scores with no change or a further decline in cognitive function in a small open-trial study.

Case Vignettes

Role Transition

Given the contribution of the field of social psychology to the development of IPT, social roles of various kinds can be understood as helping to shape the sense of identity of the patient, and conversely, changes in those roles can be seen to introduce doubts about the stability of those identity components. These doubts, when persistent, can lead to demoralization and depression.

> CASE: His daughter brought Robert for evaluation because she worried incessantly about his depressed behavior following retirement. He did not want to come but eventually gave in, and his IPT therapist was careful to first evaluate the extent of his mourning of the perceived loss of his old role or roles. Cautiously at first, Robert was able to form a working rapport with his therapist, whom he later said seemed to treat him with great respect. He seemed to resign himself to the process of IPT as he had "time on his hands and nothing better to do." Robert filled in the details of retiring after forty years of work in an industrial job as a "fixer" of mechanical problems in a repair shop. He was good at what he did and respected by his peers, and proudly described how there wasn't anything that he could not fix. Robert also loved to watch professional football games on television on weekends to root for the home team and looked forward to retirement so that he could watch as many games as he liked. In fact, Robert did enjoy the first football season after retirement but began to have second thoughts about retiring after the season ended. He missed the

guys at work and now realized that he had been important to them, and they made him feel like he belonged. He began to hate his new life of idleness, the boredom and lack of agenda after he had fixed all the household projects on his to-do list. He tried to watch daytime television but became bored and disillusioned about what retirement was really like. His daughter described that he got to the point where he sat in his finished basement with the TV and the lights off, just sitting and staring as if in a trance of depression and immobility.

As Robert and his IPT therapist continued to meet, his therapist invited him to brainstorm together about what he might try to find in his retired life that would give him some of the satisfaction he admitted getting from all the accolades he had received at work for countless jobs well done. Robert said that he had heard of a widow in their retirement complex who was in need of some help to hang shelves that he had agreed to take a look at. He admitted that he felt good about his "good deed" and guessed that he still had some value left in him. His mood began to lift and his wife could hear him whistling while he puttered in the basement setting up his tools into a workshop of sorts in one corner. As the weeks went by with continued brainstorming sessions about what he could do to make his retirement more meaningful to him, he began to offer to fix various things for other residents in his complex and became know as the "fix-it guy." He continued to refuse money for his handiwork but did oblige repeated offers to have coffee and cookies with his new neighbors and slowly began to make some new acquaintances. When it came time for termination, he was thankful for the help with "brainstorming" and felt confident that he could continue his new line of "work" for a long time to come and agreed that he did not need to meet any longer. He no longer felt depressed, and his PHQ-9 had dropped from a score of 30 to 2.

Unresolved Grief

Bereavement is the event of losing through death someone emotionally close. Losing a spouse through death can also have a component of a role transition in that roles fulfilled by the late spouse may now fall to the griever or need to be delegated elsewhere. Similarly, family dynamics can change when a death occurs, particularly the death of the family patriarch or matriarch, causing confusion or a power vacuum. In IPT for unresolved grief, considerable time is spent encouraging grievers to describe their lost loved ones, which is usually characterized soon after the death by some level of idealization as the "perfect husband, father, or provider," for example. This process can be facilitated by bringing in photographs or memorabilia to enhance and review memories. Eventually, after some weeks of idealization, there is usually some acknowledgment of annoyances or shortcomings on the part of the deceased. These too are encouraged to be "owned" and elucidated as part of a more complex and balanced picture that more accurately represents the deceased as having had a mix of endearing and not-so-endearing traits, which engenders a mix of different feelings in the griever. All of these feelings, including anger, remorse, shame, and guilt, are acknowledged to be commonly seen in the grieving process. The IPT therapist will sometimes note a flood of sad feelings that follows the recognition of annoyance or anger toward the late spouse for past transgressions or for leaving the patient without the usual support and love by dying prematurely and leaving the patient behind. Sometimes grievers need to talk about their anger toward their view of a benevolent higher power for "taking their spouse or particularly a child from them."

CASE: Grace came to IPT for depression after the death of her husband. An IPT therapist asked the griever to describe the events immediately preceding and following the death, paying particular attention to the intense feelings aroused at the time, such as guilt about secretly wishing for death to occur to end suffering on the part of the deceased, but also a reluctance about how therapy could possibly help, as nothing could bring her husband back. The interpersonal inventory revealed that she had two adult children who were married with families of their own and who both lived in distant cities. She felt close to all of them but vowed that she would never consider depending on them or moving closer to them as she could not imagine interfering with the busy lives they had. She suffered from chronic back pain and a heart arrhythmia but considered herself to be in pretty good shape otherwise and described in great detail the wonderful life she had when her husband was alive. He was a retired businessman in a medium-sized college town who was civic minded and served on several boards of charitable organizations. She too had played supporting roles that followed his initiatives, and a picture emerged of a somewhat starstruck young woman meeting the man of her dreams soon after graduating from college as a teacher. She described him as mature, steadfast, intelligent, nurturant to her, and a fine dresser. Grace went on to wistfully describe all the international trips they took together, how they had season tickets to the college sports team and "never missed a game," and how, in general, she felt proud and admired when walking arm-in-arm with him in public as "just about everyone in town knew and respected them highly."

Grace complained of no longer having anything to look forward to, as she would never consider traveling alone or going to a sporting event without him. On her worst days she felt so gloomy she wished she had just died with him, and they could have been buried side by side and thus still be together forever. She admitted wondering how she might take her own life but dismissed the idea when confronted with the thought that her husband would be very disappointed in her if she took her own life even if the reason was to be with him again.

Using nondirective exploration and clarification, Grace's IPT therapist listened intently to her descriptions of her late husband and her life before and after his death. As a theme emerged of her own identity being tightly linked to their shared life where he was something of a local celebrity, her therapist acknowledged this fact and the sadness that went with it but began to challenge her to brainstorm about ways in which she could cherish those memories but choose to "strike out on her own" and "make her own mark" on the community they both loved so much. Her therapist recognized that she was an intelligent and capable woman with many skills that had been very willingly focused on a supporting role for her husband's initiatives while he was alive but that she was eminently capable of refocusing that energy and those skills on her own chosen initiative(s). At first Grace was skeptical and felt that she could not possibly amass the respect and popular following her husband had enjoyed (with her on his arm). She struggled to brainstorm about how to make her new life feel useful and more gratifying. She surmised that other widows like herself might be having similar struggles adjusting to life without their husbands and invited two of them to meet for lunch and discuss how they might work at being supportive to each other. She worried that she might be turned down as they both had more family supports in town than she did. Grace's IPT therapist utilized decision analysis to weigh the pros and cons of acting on this plan and offered to stage a role-play exercise where she could practice how she might couch the offer to "make sure it didn't sound too maudlin." At the following session, Grace was noticeably more excited about the enthusiasm she found among the other two widows. With more brainstorming in subsequent sessions, Grace stated that she could not imagine going by herself to a theater performance like the ones she and her husband had enjoyed but would consider it fun to do so as a group and that "it would be an important new experience for the other widows," outlining the leadership role she had established for herself. Her therapist pointed out that she had successfully forged a new direction for her life that was independent of her husband and made an explicit point of linking the drop in her PHQ depression score from 30 to 5 over the course of their work together. They agreed to terminate at Session 12 as she felt she was no longer depressed and now had found a "new direction" for her life.

Role Dispute

Among the techniques utilized in IPT described earlier, role-play and communication analysis are commonly employed with a role-dispute focus to more clearly establish any discernable patterns of maladaptive or nonmutual communication.

Exploring the dispute as either at an impasse, a renegotiation stage, or the point of dissolution can help patients confront the reality of their role disputes and their own role in maintaining the status quo versus taking action to change it into something better. Once alternative strategies have been considered and the options narrowed, role-play can offer a chance to practice how to approach the other person or persons involved in the dispute to build confidence they can follow through. Attempts to try different approaches are then explored for effectiveness the following session, and adjustments are made to keep refining new strategies that work better. Any drop in depressive symptoms that results from such efforts is pointed out as clearly linked to the action taken by the identified patient, and all responsibility for newfound success is explicitly attributed to their action taking. Interpersonal psychotherapists portray themselves as merely facilitators for exploring possible options or change, and, thus, when the time comes for termination after completing the agreed upon 12–16 sessions, therapists can point out that they have confidence in patients' abilities to continue to exercise the new techniques learned in IPT on their own and thus avoid future demoralization or depression when faced with new problems or dilemmas after IPT is completed.

In some cases, particularly those with a focus on role disputes, monthly maintenance IPT is required to help remind the patient to continue to apply newly found strategies to new role disputes that arise. In contrast to those patients with an IPT focus of grief or role transition, which is likely to be resolved within the timeframe of acute IPT, those with a focus of role dispute more often fall back into their old patterns of maladaptive communication and are thus at risk for more unresolved role disputes, demoralization, and depression. Interpersonal psychotherapy is not appropriate for individuals with severe borderline personality disorders or with chronic suicidal or self-harming behaviors, as these patients show better outcomes with more intensive or structured therapies such as DBT or Intensive Outpatient Programs (IOPs).

> CASE: George presented for treatment for depression and panic attacks. He had recently moved from another city to be closer to his wife's family after he retired as a salesman for a chain store. He quickly described his life as "no picnic" living with his wife, who suffered from a seizure disorder and was often very critical of George. They had one unmarried son, who lived a long plane ride away and visited annually. George said he was looking forward to spending more time organizing his stamp collection that he was very proud of. During the move from their home to an apartment, George was frustrated by the fact that he had scant space to himself and had to keep his stamp collection under a bed instead of in a wall cupboard, as he once had in his old house. He also needed table space to sort and arrange his stamps, and he "caught hell" if he consumed more space than his wife thought proper.

George's IPT therapist suggested that a focus on role dispute seemed most appropriate with a secondary focus on role transition to retirement and moving to a new city. George agreed with this formulation and admitted that he did not mind moving to a new city or even downsizing to an apartment but stated that the increased time spent with his wife sometimes "got under his nerves." George said his wife rarely showed him much affection and would only allow him to give her a kiss on her cheek on holiday occasions when he dutifully brought her a dozen roses or other flower bouquets. He volunteered that he had given up on sexual intimacy years ago as his wife was too sickly and never seemed interested.

In the next six sessions, his IPT therapist helped him to brainstorm about how to negotiate more support from his wife and how he might stand his ground when he felt unfairly or capriciously criticized. The dispute seemed to be long-standing and engrained as a pattern that he had compensated for by escaping to work or immersing himself in his hobbies. George's IPT therapist could see that George was quite intelligent and had retired from a career where his work was far below his true capability. His main problem was poor self-esteem and panicky fear that he would die alone if his wife kicked him out such that he often waited on her hand and foot to try to appease her. He reasoned that his wife was ill with a seizure disorder and that she could not help her own temper outbursts.

George's IPT therapist used communication analysis to illustrate the imbalance of power in their relationship and facilitated brainstorming sessions about how he might take a more balanced, assertive tone and thus feel less put down by his wife despite her chronic illness. Role-play was crucial for George, who said he was not used to confronting his wife and risking more wrath from her. His attempts to consider ways to be more assertive were timid and awkward, even in role-play.

During their eighth IPT session, George sheepishly said he had something important to share that he had never told anyone: his wife occasionally hit him with her open hand and threatened when in fits of rage to destroy his stamp collection, the latter being his worst fear as he had no place to hide it from her. His IPT therapist was taken by surprise by this revelation and felt obligated to point out that this was not acceptable behavior in any relationship, which led to a discussion of George revealing that he had thought of leaving her many times but felt guilty for leaving her alone in case she had a seizure and injured herself. He was not so confident he could tolerate much more and vowed to tell her so. Another action George decided upon was to protect his stamp collection from the potential damage she threatened during her rage episodes by purchasing a metal record keeping box with a lock that was also fireproof. George's IPT therapist pointed out that despite the intensity of the emotional strain caused by this deliberate confrontation with his wife, his mood actually improved, and he said he felt good about his new path of being able to defend himself in a more assertive way when necessary. He later surmised that his wife had actually seen her neurologist as he noticed new prescription bottles of an unfamiliar medication in their apartment although he never brought it up for confirmation. He described being inwardly satisfied that she had listened to him in her own way and sought help for better control of her anger.

In the termination phase of IPT, George said he had to be realistic that his wife was not really going to change much but that he did love his wife for having chosen him over all the other men she could have picked to marry. She had saved him at the time from the worse fate of living with his mother, and he was grateful for that. The renewed hope he felt was the realization that he could take concrete steps to defend himself when he put his mind to it and take action even to the point of divorcing her if things got bad enough. He learned to leave the apartment when his wife showed raging behavior, which did decline in frequency, proclaiming to her that he would be back in several hours, hopefully when she was in a more cordial mood toward him.

This vignette illustrates that long-standing role disputes need to be assessed for a willingness to take chances and try new approaches to conquer fears. Being more assertive required him to acknowledge that such action could trigger consequences, and thus he had to be prepared mentally to back up his threat to divorce her if she could not learn to better control her rage toward him.

It is important to note that the decision to take action and the form that action would take all came from George, not his IPT therapist, who merely facilitated the brainstorming sessions, encouraged the expression of affect, helped him to analyze their respective communication styles, and facilitated his decision-making to risk-taking assertive action even if it meant filing for divorce because he had reached an impasse and was not going to tolerate physical manifestations of his wife's rage.

Interpersonal Deficit

The IPT category of interpersonal deficit is the default setting when a patient case formulation does not fit well into the other three categories. Such patients are usually more isolated and have a history of few or no mutually satisfying reciprocal relationships and, frequently, failed relationships or estrangement from family members or former supports. The strategy for helping patients with a focus of interpersonal deficit is to encourage greater interaction with others in meaningful ways that provide more social support for these aging and increasingly vulnerable individuals. In contrast to the other three foci, where the examining lens is focused on interpersonal relationships that are directly linked to their most recent depression or dysfunction, the IPT therapist utilizes the example of the patient-therapist relationship in the here-and-now as an example of a working relationship to be considered as a model for examination and experimentation. This focus is the least used in IPT, and, since such patients often have personality disorders (PDs) or traits, no short-term therapy, including IPT, would be easily capable of changing personality function. Goals for this focus in IPT are thus more limited. Helping to improve the patient's overall functioning and encouraging the establishment or maintenance of one or more supportive relationships would be considered a success, as the following case vignette will illustrate.

CASE: Ann, a 73-year-old African American female, had worked for many years as a telephone operator before retiring as soon as she could access her pension. She never married or had any children and had been estranged from the two brothers and sister she grew up with for more than 20 years, citing small, perceived slights they had committed against her. She denied being abused as a child and referred to her parents as "OK" and said she had decent clothes to wear and graduated from secretarial school after high school but did not like to type. She lived in an apartment building on a limited fixed income and stayed to herself, rarely greeting others in her building ("because you never know who will want to get into your business"). Her IPT therapist noted her past history and her tendency to use large-sized vocabulary when simpler ones would suffice, giving an odd quality to her speech. This speech peculiarity, odd color combinations in her clothing, and her theories of how the world worked had a paranoid flavor to them but nothing delusional. Overall, she showed many schizoid traits. She told her therapist she would often not talk to anyone else except the check-out clerk in a grocery store. Ann had never owned or learned how to drive a car and was content to use public transportation to get to her doctor visits. Her only entertainment besides reading and a rare television program was to attend a monthly travelogue series at a nearby museum of history where volunteers showed slideshows of international trips they had taken to exotic places. She always sat alone and never asked a question nor did she share any of her own thoughts. She never stayed for the refreshments that followed each travelogue. She self-diagnosed depression and felt that she "had it" since she was a young girl and had many questions about genetic vulnerability that she had read about. Ann said that she knew she had trouble trusting people and that she did better with professionals because they were required to be trustworthy by their professional ethics. Her IPT therapist used their therapeutic relationship to model how making casual conversation carried little risk of further unwanted expectations by talking about a few innocuous personal matters such as food, recipes, vacation visits, favorite authors, and, of course, the weather. During these role-play exercises, Ann was animated and seemed to enjoy the discussion but struggled with the idea of generalizing this discussion to other people in her real life such as possibly a neighbor in her building.

Summary

This chapter provided an overview of the basics of IPT, a relational-based brief psychotherapy, and its application to older persons who may be suffering from depression or from a combination of depression and cognitive impairment. Interpersonal psychotherapy suggests a specific structure, concentrates on relevant areas of focus, and utilizes an array of therapeutic techniques. IPT touches upon the glories and pitfalls of what makes us human: the ability to think, the ability to be creative, to feel, to problem-solve, to connect with others, to participate in social roles, and to go outside of ourselves. Interpersonal psychotherapy has proven to be an effective treatment response to these very intimate and meaningful aspects of our humanity that can be profoundly affected by depression and mild cognitive impairment.

References

1. Weissman M, Markowitz J, Klerman G. *Comprehensive guide to interpersonal psychotherapy.* New York: Basic Books; 2000.

2. Weissman M, Markowitz J, Klerman G. *The guide to interpersonal psychotherapy.* New York: Oxford University Press; 2018.

3. Bruce M, Ten Have RL, Reynolds T III, et al. Reducing suicidal ideation and depressive symptoms in depressed older primary care patients. *JAMA.* 2004;291 (9):1081.

4. Unützer J, Katon W, Callahan C, et al. Collaborative care management of late-life depression in the primary care setting. *JAMA.* 2002;288(22):2836.

5. Miller MD, Wolfson LK, Frank E, et al. Using interpersonal psychotherapy (IPT) in a combined psychotherapy/ medication research protocol with depressed elders. *J Psychother Pract Res.* 1998;7:47–55.

6. Van Hees ML, Rotter T, Ellerman T, Evers SM. The effectiveness of individual interpersonal psychotherapy as a treatment for major depressive disorder in adult outpatients: a systematic review. *Biomed Central Psychiatry.* 2013;13:22.

7. DeMello MF, Mari JJ, Baclachuk J, et al. A systematic review of research findings on the efficacy of interpersonal psychotherapy for depressive disorders. *Eur Arch Psychiatry Clin Neurosci.* 2005;255:75–82.

8. van Schaik DJ, van Marwijk HW, Beekman AT. Interpersonal psychotherapy (IPT) for late-life depression in general practice: uptake and satisfaction by patients, therapists and physicians. *BMC Family Practice.* 2007;8:52.

9. Post EP, Miller MD, Schulberg HC. Using interpersonal psychotherapy (IPT) to treat

depression in older primary care patients. *Geriatrics*. 2008; 63(3):18–28.

10. Miller MD, Frank E, Cornes C. Applying interpersonal psychotherapy to bereavement-related depression following loss of a spouse in late life. *J Psychother Pract Res*. 1994;32:149–162.

11. Reynolds CF, Miller MD, Pasternak RE. Treatment of bereavement-related major depressive episodes in later life: a controlled study of acute and continuation treatment with nortriptyline and interpersonal psychotherapy. *Am J Psychiatry*. 1999;15:202–208.

12. Elkin I, Shea MT, Watkins JT, et al. National institute of mental health treatment of depression collaborative research program. General effectiveness of treatments. *Arch Gen Psychiatry*. 1989;53 (10):913–919.

13. Reynolds C 3rd, Frank E, Perel J, et al. Nortriptyline and interpersonal psychotherapy as maintenance therapies for recurrent major depression: a randomized controlled trial in patients older than fifty-nine years. *JAMA*. 1999;281 (1):39–45.

14. Miller MD, Frank E, Cornes C. The value of maintenance interpersonal psychotherapy (IPT) in older adults with different IPT foci. *Am J Geriatr Psychiatry* 2003;10:1–6.

15. Reynolds, C 3rd, Dew M, Pollock B, et al. Maintenance treatment of depression in old age. *New England Journal of Medicine*. 2006;354(23):1130–1138.

16. Carreira K, Miller MD, Frank E, et al. A controlled evaluation of monthly maintenance interpersonal psychotherapy in late-life depression with varying levels of cognitive function. *Int J Geriatr Psychiatry*. 2008;23;1110–1113.

17. Reynolds CF, Dew MA, Martire LM. Treating depression to remission in older adults: a controlled evaluation of combined escitalopram with interpersonal psychotherapy vs. escitalopram with depression care management. *Int J Geriatr Psychiatry*. 2010;25 (11):1134–1141.

18. Arean PA, Cook BL. Psychotherapy and combined psychotherapy/ pharmacotherapy for late life depression. *Biological Psychiatry*. 2002;52(3): 293–303.

19. Taylor MP, Reynolds CF, Frank E, et al. Which elderly depressed patients remain well on maintenance interpersonal psychotherapy alone? report from the Pittsburgh study of maintenance therapies in late-life depression. *Depress Anxiety*. 1999;10:55–60.

20. Miller MD, Richards V, Zukoff A, et al. A model for modifying interpersonal psychotherapy (IPT) for depressed elders with cognitive impairment. *Clin Gerontol*. 2006;30(2):79–101.

21. Miller MD, Reynolds CF. Expanding the usefulness of interpersonal psychotherapy (IPT) for depressed elders with co-morbid cognitive impairment. *Int J Geriatr Psychiatry*. 2007;22:101–105.

22. Miller M. *Clinician's guide to interpersonal psychotherapy in late life*. New York: Oxford University Press; 2009.

23. Nasreddine ZS, Phillips NA, Bediran V. The Montreal cognitive assessment, MOCA: a brief screening tool for mild cognitive impairment. *J Am Geriatr Soc*. 2005;53(4):695–699.

24. Kroenke K, Spitzer, J.B. Williams. The PHQ-9: validity of a brief depression measure. *J Gen Intern Med*. 2001;16 (9):606–613.

Chapter

7

Short-Term Psychodynamic Psychotherapy

Patricia Coughlin and Brandon C. Yarns

Introduction

Short-term psychodynamic psychotherapy (STPP) is an evidence-based treatment modality for older adults.[1] Similar to cognitive behavioral therapy (CBT),[2] STPP refers to a family of distinct but overlapping therapies that share similar features.[3,4] All STPP modalities are rooted in psychoanalytic theory and share the notion that unconscious emotional conflicts are largely responsible for our patients' symptoms and suffering.[5]

In a seminal study, STPP was easily distinguished from CBT based on three key differences: (1) a focus on affective experience, emphasizing the importance of bringing troublesome feelings into awareness; (2) linking current conflicts and difficulties with unresolved conflicts from the past; and (3) using the therapist-patient relationship as a change agent.[6] STPP may be performed in group or individual settings.[3]

Evidence Base for STPP with Older Adults

The Society for Clinical Psychology, Division 12 of the American Psychological Association, lists STPP as an evidence-based treatment for depression, including for geriatric depression.[7] Several positive clinical trials support the use of STPP in older adults. In a randomized sample of 33 depressed older adults, 20 completed nine months of treatment with either CBT or psychodynamic group treatment; no clinically significant differences were found posttreatment, based on *a priori* criteria for clinical significance, but a statistically significant difference was found favoring CBT on the Beck Depression Inventory (BDI).[8]

In a separate trial, 91 elders with major depressive disorder (MDD) received 16–20 sessions of cognitive, behavioral, or structured STPP with no differences in outcomes at posttreatment[9] or at 2-year follow-up.[10] The authors concluded that one key to the success of STPP used in this trial was the structured (versus unstructured) format.[10] Finally, the same group randomized 66 depressed caregivers to 20 sessions of either CBT or STPP; no differences in any outcome were found at posttreatment, although duration of caregiving predicted preferential treatment response with shorter caregiving duration favoring STPP and longer caregiving duration favoring CBT.[11]

Several recent meta-analyses included the above trials and reported benefits of STPP for late-life depression.[12–14] In addition, a meta-analysis of psychotherapy for depression among patients with Parkinson's disease presented interesting findings that STPP outperformed CBT in nine different comparative effectiveness trials in this population, mostly conducted in China.[15]

Intensive Short-Term Dynamic Psychotherapy

The authors have significant clinical experience using an experiential form of STPP in older adults called intensive short-term dynamic psychotherapy (ISTDP), and one author (BCY) is currently conducting a clinical trial using elements of ISTDP in a group format called emotional awareness and expression therapy (EAET)[16-18] for older adults with chronic musculoskeletal pain compared to CBT for chronic pain (CBT-CP). At the time of this writing, N = 24 older adults have been randomized to the ISTDP-based condition and N = 24 to CBT, and N = 35 have completed treatment with experts in the treatment condition to which they have been randomly assigned. Whereas differences between patient satisfaction with treatment and dropout rates were small and similar between the 2 groups, a nonsignificant trend toward more improvement in the primary outcome of posttreatment pain severity was found which favored the ISTDP-based treatment over CBT (t = 1.868, p = 0.07). In fact, several patients in the ISTDP-based condition (N = 3, 18%) had large improvements in pain severity, greater than -3 on an 11-point (0–10) scale, whereas no patient in the CBT condition had such large improvements. Overall, the ISTDP-based condition delivered a moderate effect size of -0.60 for pain severity, whereas CBT had a small effect size of -0.22. Additional groups are planned, and secondary outcome data, as well as 3-month follow-up data, from these participants are currently being analyzed. These tentative and preliminary findings indicate that an ISTDP-based treatment is a reasonable alternative to CBT for older adults with chronic musculoskeletal pain, and may turn out to be more efficacious in this population.

Intensive Short-Term Dynamic Psychotherapy Metapsychology

Metapsychology refers to the overarching psychological theory on which a particular psychotherapy modality is based.[19] Developed by Habib Davanloo from the 1970s to the early 2000s, ISTDP is a psychoanalytically-oriented psychotherapy based upon Freud's Second Theory of Anxiety.[20-23] Freud's theoretical shift was, in many ways, the beginning of an attachment theory, viewing anxiety as a signal that any thought, feeling, or fantasy that could threaten the bond with caretakers was dangerous and must be avoided. Defenses are used to accomplish this end. While serving an adaptive function in childhood, defenses often outlive their usefulness and actually create the problems and symptoms the adult is experiencing. For example, learning to suppress anger by putting on a happy face and becoming pleasing and compliant may secure the child's relationship with a demanding parent. However, the habitual suppression of anger often leads to depression and fatigue, while the perpetuation of a compliant, submissive stand regarding the wishes of others almost insures chronic resentment and the perpetuation of unmet needs.

In cases where frustration in and rupture to the attachment bond is severe or repetitive, and there is no repair or support for the powerful feelings generated thereby, **attachment trauma** can result, and more severe psychopathology often follows. Bowlby has suggested that children develop murderous rage in response to such attachment trauma.[24] When the child experiences murderous rage toward those he needs and loves, profound guilt is generated. Defenses against these guilt-laden feelings and wishes often create a self-destructive system in which the child either punishes the self (e.g., withdrawal and isolation, cutting, and anorexia) or invites others to do so. Without intervention, symptoms such as depression, self-imposed isolation, and a lifelong pattern of self-sabotage can result.[22,25] The hypothesized cascade of feelings that occurs in response to unprocessed attachment trauma

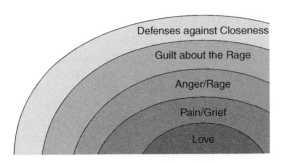

Figure 7.1 Attachment Feelings

is shown in Figure 7.1, with the outermost circle indicating the development of defensive isolation in response to the avoidance of these feelings.

Davanloo has suggested that the only way to cure symptoms and return the patient to psychological health is to help him relinquish defenses in order to face and experience his "true feelings about the past and the present."[22] He discovered that the visceral experience of previously avoided feelings was the trigger that "unlocked" the unconscious. This unlocking produces a download of memories, shedding light on the origin of the patient's emotional conflicts. In this way, the past becomes vividly present and is available for reworking. Neuroscientific evidence on state-dependent learning and memory reconsolidation[26,27] has supported Davanloo's clinical findings in this regard. The experience and healthy expression of painful and conflictual feelings is the key to unlocking both the unconscious source of the patient's suffering and the patient's innate healing force (which Davanloo refers to as the **unconscious therapeutic alliance**).

While the CBT therapist helps the patient modify conscious thoughts and behaviors in order to decrease painful feelings, the ISTDP therapist helps the patient abandon defenses and experience painful feelings, in order to uncover the unconscious source of his suffering. There is accumulating evidence to suggest that the bulk of our patients' symptoms and difficulties resides in unconscious, implicit emotional learnings.[26,27] Intensive short-term dynamic psychotherapy has proven an effective method of unearthing the unconscious source of suffering, as well as facilitating healing and recovery. In addition, long-term follow-up demonstrates that the therapeutic effects obtained in ISTDP treatment are not only maintained over time but actually increase with no further treatment.[28,29] This is in contrast to most therapies, including CBT,[30,31] that have large relapse rates of up to 60–65% over five years.

Feelings, Anxiety, and Defense, and the Two Triangles

Intensive short-term dynamic psychotherapists use Two Triangles to guide the therapeutic process. Figure 7.2 displays the Two Triangles.

The **Triangle of Conflict** (on the left in Figure 7.2), developed by Karl Menninger, depicts the relationship between the patient's feelings and impulses, anxiety, and defenses.[32] David Malan, an expert on STPP, added the **Triangle of Persons** (on the right in Figure 7.2) in order to represent the interpersonal nature of our emotional conflicts.[33] When we link the two triangles together, we can understand the original source of the patient's conflict, as well as see how these unresolved conflicts from the past can be repeated in the patient's current life and are often apparent in interactions with the therapist, where they can be experienced and modified in real time. These triangles help the dynamic therapist

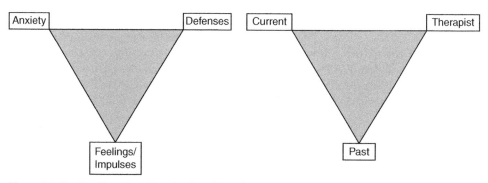

Figure 7.2 The Two Triangles – Triangle of Conflict (Left) and Triangle of Persons (Right).

understand the material being presented, as well as guide her interventions. In order to be consistently effective, the therapist must constantly monitor all six corners of the Two Triangles. For now, we will elaborate further on the three corners of the Triangle of Conflict.

Feelings

Feelings are discrete, internal experiences of arousal associated with specific action tendencies, or impulses.[34,35] These feelings and impulses have been selected for in evolution,[36] providing us with energy and important information from within. They help us prioritize, make decisions, and connect deeply with others.

When patients habitually defend against these feelings, they suffer emotionally, physically, interpersonally, and occupationally.[37,38] Therefore, one of the central tasks of ISTDP is to facilitate the patient's ability to experience the full range of human feelings. In particular, feelings that are suffused with anxiety and chronically avoided must be faced and experienced in order to facilitate health and healing.[29,39]

Davanloo has developed an operational definition of what is meant by being "in touch with feelings." He suggested that three key components must be present: (1) **a cognitive label**, (2) **physiological activation** consistent with the stated affect, and (3) **mobilization of the accompanying impulse or action tendency**.[20] The cognitive component refers to the ability to correctly identify and label the feeling being experienced. For example, the patient is able to say, "I feel really angry with my husband for forgetting my birthday." This connotes cognitive clarity. The physiological component refers to the somatic manifestations of the emotion identified. If we stay with the example of anger, we would expect to see an increase in heat, energy, and strength, originating in the gut or chest and spreading into the limbs, neck, and jaw.[25] Finally, feelings are important because what we *feel* in a given situation gives us information from within about what we need to *do* in that situation.[36] This is known as the behavioral component of the feeling, the action tendency, or the impulse. The physiological activation of anger triggers an impulse to defend ourselves and our loved ones, establish boundaries, and set limits. Aggressive impulses to punch, kick, bite, and even kill a perpetrator or intruder are mobilized when rage is experienced.[25] It is important to note that, in ISTDP, we seek to facilitate the full experience of all of the patient's mixed feelings, rather than just one discrete affect. (See Figure 7.1 and the first Case Example below.)

Anxiety

According to Freud's Second Theory of Anxiety, anxiety is a *signal* that painful and conflictual feelings are being aroused and are threatening to come into consciousness.[20,21] According to Davanloo, there are three distinct channels of anxiety, each with diagnostic significance. These are: (1) **striated or voluntary muscle anxiety**, (2) **smooth or involuntary muscle activation**, and (3) **cognitive-perceptual disruption (CPD)**.[20,22,23] Striated muscle anxiety refers to anxiety that results in tension of voluntary skeletal muscles, such as sighing respirations, hand clenching, or foot tapping.[25] Patients who are able to bind their anxiety in muscle tension are typically aware that they are anxious and have some idea what has triggered the anxiety, suggesting a fairly high **ego adaptive capacity**. Activation of smooth, involuntary muscles, including those in the blood vessels and gut, may result in exacerbations of serious medical conditions like hypertension, irritable bowel syndrome, ulcerative colitis, and migraine headaches.[25,40] Patients who rely on this pathway of discharge are often consciously *un*aware of their anxiety and its effect on their physical health. Finally, CPD refers to anxiety that disrupts the patient's *cognitions*, with manifestations such as mental confusion, memory lapses, or dissociation, and/or the patient's *perceptions*, with manifestations such as blurry vision or tinnitus.[25] An individual patient may manifest any or all of the three channels of anxiety, depending on the level and intensity of the anxiety and the underlying feelings triggering it.

Assessing and regulating anxiety, in order to intervene within the window of the patient's anxiety tolerance, is essential for the effective implementation of intensive short-term dynamic psychotherapy. Anxiety is our safety gauge. It is only safe to explore the experience of anxiety-provoking feelings and wishes when patients are able to experience anxiety in their striated or voluntary muscles. Specific interventions designed to build anxiety tolerance are required for the safe and effective use of ISTDP in patients who originally present with smooth muscle involvement or cognitive-perceptual disruption. This is common sense; we cannot engage in collaborative psychotherapy with patients who are dissociating or experiencing migraine headaches in the session! Conversely, patients who are detached and uninvolved, experiencing no anxiety, are unlikely to benefit from treatment. Optimal levels of anxiety are necessary for new learning and growth,[41,42] so a constant monitoring of anxiety is crucial in achieving positive therapeutic outcomes.

Defenses

Since it is the patient's excessive reliance on defenses that create and perpetuate his suffering, helping the patient become aware of, and then relinquishing, defenses is necessary to facilitate healing. Davanloo has described two classes of defenses: **formal defenses** and **tactical defenses**.[20,22] Formal defenses,[43] like rationalization, projection, and somatization, serve the dual purposes of lowering anxiety and preventing painful feelings from coming into conscious awareness. The type of defenses typically employed by a given patient reveals important diagnostic information regarding the patient's level of ego adaptive capacity.[20,22,44] Those who rely on repressive, intellectualizing defenses have the ability to "mentalize" or think about feelings, while those who rely on regressive defenses lack this essential function. Consequently, these categories of patients require different types of intervention.

In addition to the formal defenses we are all familiar with, Davanloo has identified another group of defenses he has referred to as "tactical defenses."[22] While formal defenses are used to prevent the patient from experiencing anxiety-provoking feelings internally, tactical defenses are employed interpersonally. Since our feelings are triggered by close contact with others, if we cannot tolerate such feelings, we will have to keep others at a distance. When a caring person, like a therapist, attempts to enter the intimate, emotional life of the patient, all the feelings regarding past failed relationships tend to be evoked (see Figure 7.1). Defenses against these feelings become a resistance to closeness in the therapeutic relationship. Such defenses can take both verbal (being vague and general, contradicting oneself, being sarcastic and defiant) and nonverbal forms (avoiding eye contact, crossing arms and legs). If unaddressed, these tactical defenses create a barrier to the very kind of emotional connection required for successful treatment. Unless the therapist is skilled in identifying and challenging these tactical defenses, the therapy will remain superficial and fail to address the underlying cause of the patient's disturbance.

Davanloo has developed a systematic and structured method for assessing the nature and tenacity of defenses, as well as outlining an effective method for removing them.[22,45] The process involves: (1) identification of the defense, (2) clarification of the function of the defense, and (3) examination of the cost of the defense. For example, when asking about feelings toward a critical boss, a depressed patient typically responds with something like, "I guess I deserved it. I am a lousy employee." The therapist needs to *identify* the defense in operation: "That is a criticism of you, not a feeling toward your boss. What was your feeling toward your boss for criticizing you in front of the whole team?" Once the patient can see that she is avoiding the feeling with the use of a defense, we *clarify the function* of the defense. The therapist might say, "That is the way you avoid the feeling toward him – by turning it back on yourself." The patient must be able to see that she is *doing something* to avoid her feelings. If the patient is highly identified with her defenses, she might say something like, "That's the way I do anger. When I am angry, I cry." In such cases, it may take several repetitions for the patient to be able to make the distinction between her feelings and the defenses against them. Once that distinction is clear, we can move on to an *examination of the cost* of the defense. If we stay with our example, we would ask, "What happens when you do that – when you turn your anger toward others back on yourself with self-attack and collapse into tears?" Can the patient see that the defense of internalization creates and perpetuates depression? This is a crucial step in the process of defense work, and is necessary for the patient to turn on the defenses that hurt her. Once the patient sees the operation of the defense and how it causes her problems, she is in a position to make a conscious decision about whether to continue to avoid these feelings or to face them honestly, in the service of healing.

The Central Dynamic Sequence

Intensive short-term dynamic psychotherapy involves a systematic but flexible approach to treatment, based on the needs and capacities of each patient. Since developmental history and DSM diagnoses fail to provide us with information about the underlying *causes* of a patient's difficulties, they cannot guide us in the selection of a treatment strategy to address the source of the problem. Davanloo has urged us to use "response to intervention" as the most timely and accurate data about the nature of the underlying conflicts responsible for patients' symptoms and suffering, as well as their capacity to tolerate the emotional upheaval involved in the process of psychotherapy.[20,22,45]

The structure of an ISTDP session is outlined in what Davanloo called the **Central Dynamic Sequence (CDS)**.[46] The CDS involves a series of phases, beginning with a specific and detailed inquiry into the nature, history, and severity of the presenting complaints. The process moves to an assessment and regulation of anxiety as well as an identification and removal of defenses in order to help patients face and experience the feelings they have been avoiding. Following this breakthrough of painful feelings into awareness, memories regarding the origin of patients' emotional conflict are derepressed and processed.[20,46] Such memories supply the information we need to understand the origin of patients' conflicts.

Implementing the CDS, and tracking patients' responses to each phase of the process, takes time. Davanloo suggested allowing at least three hours for this initial evaluation, also referred to as a **trial therapy**.[47,48] He has found that doing so accelerates and condenses the therapeutic process. Research supports the idea that spending an extended period of time in the initial session enhances outcome.[44] In contrast to a traditional psychiatric interview, research suggests that implementing the CDS in the first session yields impressive results, with one-third of all patients needing no further help at six-week follow-up.[49–53]

Special Considerations in Performing Intensive Short-Term Dynamic Psychotherapy with Older Adults

Given the conventional wisdom – that psychotherapy with older adults must be slow and limited to the attainment of only modest goals – some readers may be surprised that we advocate a rapid and intensive psychodynamic approach for our older patients. After all, Freud assumed that effective psychoanalysis could not be performed on patients beyond age thirty-five! Yet recent neuroscience research shows that older adults can continue to learn, since brain growth and development, including increases in synapses and dendritic spines – and even growth of new neurons – can continue into old age with sufficient psychosocial stimulation.[54–56]

Research also suggests that being in a crisis is a positive prognostic factor for doing penetrating work in a brief amount of time.[33] Facing illness and death can precipitate just such a crisis and provide motivation for older patients to have an honest look at how they have lived their lives. In our clinical experience, significant and lasting change can take place rapidly with many older patients. Therefore, we caution against the prejudice that *all* older adults are "set in their ways" and unable to make deep and substantive change in therapy.

We have found several particular issues that frequently arise with older adults engaging in intensive short-term dynamic psychotherapy. First, an assessment of the older adult's current capacity for ISTDP is of critical importance. In particular, the ISTDP therapist must have sufficient skill to sort out what is anxiety, what is resistance, and what is cognitive impairment (CI). Although brief cognitive screening instruments such as the Mini-Mental State Examination[57] or the Montreal Cognitive Assessment (MoCA)[58] may be useful, we have found that they are often influenced negatively by anxiety in the form of cognitive-perceptual disruption. Davanloo has suggested that capacity can best be assessed through the therapist's moment-to-moment monitoring of the patient's response to intervention.[22,44] In this way, the therapist can assess the impact that anxiety and defenses have on cognitive functioning.

Additionally, older patients may be referred by others, such as a family member or physician, rather than self-referred. Effective therapists must be adept at assessing and activating the patient's own motivation and desire for change. These challenges will be further explored in the case examples that follow.

Length of Treatment

Intensive short-term dynamic psychotherapy and other forms of STPP are accelerated psychodynamic treatment and considerably shorter than long-term psychodynamic therapy or psychoanalysis. Many forms of STPP used in research protocols are time limited. However, ISTDP sets no artificial time limit but provides interventions designed to help the clinician intervene as effectively and efficiently as possible. Therapeutic results can be obtained in as few as two to three sessions but can extend as long as 50–60 sessions for more impaired patients.

Case Examples

The following cases will illustrate the application of ISTDP with two older patients. Both had life-long histories of psychiatric symptoms, unexplained pain and medical symptoms, and significant interpersonal difficulties, and had been referred by their physicians. In each case, the patients had failed to improve in numerous psychotherapy and medication trials. In contrast, both patients achieved both symptom relief and major improvement in functioning following a short course of intensive short-term dynamic psychotherapy. It is our contention that specific techniques, used to address specific problems in affective awareness and integration, were largely responsible for achieving these ends.

Case #1 The Woman Who Thought It Was Too Late

This 69-year-old single woman was referred for psychotherapy by her primary physician. The patient called incessantly and visited her physician weekly, demanding help with a host of vague complaints, none of which was found to have a medical cause. Her physician reported, "I have never had a coherent conversation with her. She is scattered and tangential, so I can't make heads or tails of what she is trying to communicate. I don't know if she is demented or has a mental illness, but I am desperate. Can you see her?" The patient was long-retired from teaching, had no close friends, and led an isolated existence. What follows is the opening interchange of the first session:

THERAPIST (TH): Why don't you start by telling me what brings you and what kind of help you are looking for?

PATIENT (PT): I don't know. I think I have to decide. This is the problem – and I do have a close friend I talk to about this. I may be – uh – I have sat – uh – all my life and because of anxiety – she feels – and I asked her because she knows me since graduate school – a lack of self-esteem, anxiety, inability to make a decision. I just sit and I really haven't gotten any... I think it's too late to get where I want to get at 69, so I go through a little anger about this nastiness about being an old maid.

This opening statement was, in fact, quite incoherent. Her facial expressions communicated exasperation and utter contempt for the process. The first task was to determine whether her incoherent pattern of speech and bizarre facial expressions were the result of high anxiety, the use of primitive defenses, or some organic disease process.

TH: So, let's just slow down and look at what you're saying so far. You are aware that you have quite a lot of anxiety and you can get paralyzed in the face of it, so that you are not able to make decisions that are in your own best interest. It also sounds like you have started to give up on yourself, saying, "It's too late; I'm 69."

PT: I am starting to – I'm sorry – I didn't mean to interrupt – I am very, my mind. . . I may be ADD. I hope I am going to remember this.

This is very important information. The patient revealed that her anxiety was so high that she was not able to focus or concentrate on the task at hand. The therapist needed to help the patient downregulate her anxiety, to see if her mental slippage improved. If so, that would suggest that anxiety, rather than dementia, was responsible for her cognitive dysfunction.

To help her regulate anxiety, the therapist suggested she focus her attention on the bodily signals of distress, rather than her scattered thoughts. Patients cannot regulate anxiety they are not aware of, so focusing attention on the bodily signals of anxiety is both diagnostic and potentially therapeutic. This type of intervention can be viewed as an experiment. Again, only patients' responses to intervention will give us the diagnostic information we need to proceed.

TH: You mentioned anxiety as a problem. Now you are saying you have difficulty focusing and being clear in your thoughts. I'm glad you let me know that. Let's slow down so we can really look at how you are experiencing this anxiety in your body. What is happening inside that lets you know you are anxious?

PT: Everything starts going around like this. (motioning to her head swirling)

TH: What else do you experience with the anxiety? What is actually happening in your body that lets you know you are anxious, nervous?

PT: It's just spinning up here in my head.

TH: So, you don't allow yourself to experience the anxiety in a bodily way – it goes up into your head and your thoughts? (indicating cognitive disruption)

PT: Maybe I do because one of my major problems is back pain. I get so tight. (This is a positive sign of striated muscle activation.)

TH: OK, that's important. So, are you willing to actually pay attention to yourself and to focus – to see if you have tension in your body, and if so, where? Do you feel any up here right now? Let's just scan your body and see.

PT: See this is a test, and I'm going to fail it.

In this vignette, the patient was able to focus her attention on anxiety in such a way that she decreased its intensity. As the anxiety was lowered, her confusion cleared up, and she was able to detect muscle tension in the back. However, high and unregulated anxiety was not the only barrier to therapeutic engagement. Once her cognition cleared up, the entrenched character defenses of hopelessness and helplessness came into view. ("See this is a test, and I'm going to fail it.") Unaddressed, such malignant character defenses would prevent the development of a therapeutic alliance so essential for effective psychotherapy. The therapeutic focus must shift from anxiety regulation to defense work.

TH: Are you interested in looking at the way you relate to yourself?

PT: Um-hum.

TH: A part of you comes here to look at some debilitating difficulties, but this other part of you is already telling you, "Don't bother. You can't succeed anyway." This is a mean way of treating yourself, hum? Do you see that? Can we put that critical voice . . .?

PT: I have been working on myself, plus everybody else. (doesn't actually answer the question)

TH: But do you see that? The way you are relating to yourself? And then also, in a sense, from the very beginning, how you are inviting me to treat you?

PT: I don't know.

TH: Well, let's look at that, because we are having a conversation, but you are wanting to turn it into a test that you are going to fail. What kind of way is that to treat you and what does that set me up as, from the get-go? (examining the transference pattern of behavior as soon as it manifests itself)

PT: Because I really can't do it.

TH: If you could, you wouldn't be here, right?

PT: I can't do anything.

TH: Let's not exaggerate. You got yourself here, right? So, let's slow down and see what's happening inside. You've got a lot of anxiety and it's almost like you are afraid to even hope that you might be able to get some help. Instead, you have this tendency to put yourself down and go hopeless. What kind of way is that to live? You must get depressed, too.

PT: (Big sigh).

The therapist identified the defenses of hopelessness and helplessness, while encouraging the patient to examine their attendant costs. By highlighting the patient's conflict between the part of her that wants help with the part that could defeat our efforts, the conflict was intensified. She responded with a heavy sigh, indicating that her anxiety was now in striated muscles, where it would be safe to examine her underlying feelings. In addition, the downregulation of her anxiety resulted in cognitive clarity. The scattered, incoherent speech evident at the start of the interview was no longer present. In addition, the work on defenses increased her willingness to participate in the process in an open and honest fashion.

TH: What are you feeling right now? Do you notice those sighs?

PT: All of the sudden I felt this whole area (middle of her body, as well as arms, shoulders, and neck).

TH: Great. What did you feel in there?

PT: I am tight up here (arms, shoulders, and neck).

TH: There is this tightness and anxiety and a lot of feelings underneath.

PT: Yes, I get very angry.

TH: How do you experience this anger inside?

PT: I just feel tight in here (arms, shoulders, and neck).

TH: It's like, right under this anxiety, there is a lot of anger that starts to come up.

PT: Yes.

TH: How do you feel it inside?

PT: It's like heat and energy.

TH: And if that anger came up and out, here, against me, what do you see, what do you want to do?

As her anxiety was downregulated and her defenses were removed, underlying feelings of pent-up anger were revealed. By encouraging her to face these feelings directly toward the therapist, we hoped to gain direct access to the source of her suffering. In so doing, we could also pave the way for a healing relationship, rather than recreating another failed relationship.

PT: Start hollering at you like, "Why am I here and you can't help me? Why am I here – and what is – why are you? You don't get it. You don't get it."

TH: So, the words don't quite make it. There is this vicious anger inside you.

PT: Yeah, I can get very angry.

TH: And if that got let loose, this animal part of you came out at me. What is in your body that wants to come out with this pent-up rage? In your imagination, if you lost control and all this tremendous rage came out toward me . . .

PT: I'd probably flip you over. Maybe slam some lamps around.

TH: You're not angry with the lamps but with me, so it would be to slam me around, huh?

PT: Right, yes. I would just take your legs and just bash you into the wall with your legs.

TH: What else?

PT: Stomp on your head.

TH: I am down and you stomp on me.

PT: Yes, and then I stomp on your torso.

TH: What else, if all this came out?

PT: Bite you in your face. Rip your arms out. Smack you. Kick you.

TH: So, it is biting, kicking, smashing me – a massive attack, on me, on my head, on my torso. Anything else in you that wants to come out at me?

PT: No, that's the problem. I think I remember biting in the third or fourth grade.

TH: So, you have had this rage almost all your life, right?

PT: Yes.

TH: So, in your imagination, when all that rage is out, my head is smashed, you bite my face, you have kicked me, stomped me, what do I look like? What is the picture?

Helping patients to experience, rather than avoid, their reactive anger about attachment failures is just the start of the process. We do not want to stop there, but help them to access, tolerate, and integrate all their mixed feelings toward caretakers, which we do by asking for the damage inflicted by the patient's rage. ("What do I look like? What is the picture?") This woman had little difficulty in acknowledging primitive rage. Connecting with the deeper feelings of pain, guilt, and love (see Figure 7.1) was more difficult – but required to facilitate healing. In the following sequence, interventions designed to help her face these mixed feelings directly were employed.

PT: You're broken. You are lying there. You are not moving. You are not talking, thank God. And I leave you.

TH: OK, but before you do that (encouraging patient to stick with it rather than avoid difficult feelings), how do I look when you are done with me?

PT: You are not moving. Your head is smashed.

TH: Am I dead?

PT: Yeah!

TH: What do you see?

PT: I just see you lying on the floor. Your head is down.

TH: And if you rolled me over and look into my face?

PT: You are just – your eyes are rolled up into your head, like dead people. Your mouth would fall open and maybe I'd just step on you a couple more times.

TH: So, there is more anger?

PT: Cause I can't have you to beat anymore. It's no fun to kick a dead body.

TH: Kind of futile, huh? So, then what is the feeling after all this rage is out? What is the feeling?

PT: I guess I'm leaving but I don't know where I'm going.

TH: But what is the feeling toward me once the rage is out?

PT: I don't care about you. Why should I care about you? Why, when no one cares about me or ever has? I've cared – see, that's the problem. I have cared too fucking much about people and I always get left in the lurch.

TH: So, you have had a lot of pain and a lot of rage inside and don't want to let anybody get close enough to activate these feelings. Where does that leave you then? You destroy me and there is no possibility. And then you leave – *by yourself* again. And even though you try to convince yourself that you don't care, what we see underneath is a lot of pain. A lot of grief. You actually do care.

PT: I don't care. Finally, this is the first time that I just care about myself! The first time.

TH: What's it like to live, only caring for yourself? What kind of life is that?

PT: Lately I've been living – it's brittle and dry.

TH: Not much of a solution huh?

PT: No.

TH: So, when you said, I don't want to care about you. Nobody cared about me. You don't even know me – so who were you talking to? Who are you so angry with? Who hurt you so badly that you just want to kill them, stomp on them?

PT: I don't know that she hurt me, but I just absolutely adored my mother and she was always so fucking busy and she was so nervous. People would never know this. Everyone loved my mother. Loved her. (crying)

This sequence reflects the ISTDP therapist's persistent attempts to reach the real, live human being stuck beneath the layers of defense and resistance that had been built up over decades. Underneath her defiant and contemptuous stance was a deep well of rage and grief regarding attachment failures. Whenever a new caregiver entered her life, all of her repressed longings, rage, grief, and guilt got activated and triggered high anxiety and destructive defenses that, left unaddressed, created a resistance to treatment. In ISTDP, these defenses were challenged as soon as they appeared. Simultaneously, the patient was encouraged to connect with and reveal her underlying feelings. The breakdown of defenses and breakthrough of feelings created an opening in which a genuine therapeutic alliance could be developed. In addition, this opening provided memories and associations (to her relationship with her mother) that shed light on the origin of the patient's problems. In this way, she could be helped to face and resolve old conflicts, rather than repeat them in her current life.

Immediately following this first session, the referring physician called to say, "I don't know what you did, but the patient and I had our first coherent conversation today. She was downright pleasant!" After four sessions, the patient reported a significant decrease in anxiety, depression, and hopelessness, with an increase in well-being. She reconnected with her love of art and the French language, taking trips to New York City to visit museums, and then becoming a docent herself! By her own report, she had never been invited to experience and express her anxiety-provoking feelings in therapy. She felt this was a crucial first step in her recovery. No longer afraid of her own intense feelings, and no longer scaring others away with her chronic use of primitive defenses, she was free to create a fulfilling life at long last.

Case #2 The Man Addicted to Pornography

This 65-year-old married attorney was referred for individual psychotherapy when couples therapy came to an end. He had had many previous attempts at therapy, as well as 12-step programs, none of which resulted in therapeutic change.

TH: Tell me what brings you and how I can help.

PT: What started it was – my wife was concerned about the Percocet (for back pain), but then what really got me into hot water was – I have had a fixation for years, since age 11, on pornography, which started to focus on fetish photos of ladies in boots and all the BDSM kind of photography. And, in later years, it's just been a fetish of, hum, ah, uh, though there were times years ago – we've been married for 24 years – but there was a period a few years ago, between 10 and 5 years ago, a little bit of dabbling near the fringe with ladies – I am not proud, but –

TH: So, your wife is concerned, but what is your concern about it?

PT: I'm not anguished over it, but this is serious stuff for me. *She* is a serious issue for me.

TH: It doesn't concern you?

PT: Only in so far as, I am not going to let this take my wife.

TH: So, this behavior is destructive: It could destroy your relationship with her. You don't see that it is destructive to you. So, the issue is, do you want to get to the bottom of this? To what is driving this self-destructive behavior that could destroy a very good marriage of 24 years?

PT: Yeah, I think I should. I'll tell you why. Now I am in a period – she laid the law down when she saw that I was doing it again. That was six weeks ago, and I promised her I won't do it and I haven't done it since then, but I see the behavior as addictive and, being an addict – I know, I deal with addicts every day – with addictive behavior, you go back to it.

TH: Unless you get to the bottom of it, to what is driving it and what you're avoiding by distracting yourself.

PT: Maybe there is a related issue. I have always been with this – on the one hand, this obsessive sex drive but, on the other hand, almost squeamish about having sex, and it disturbs me because I am married to a girl who is cute as a button. She is 55 years old and probably the cutest 55-year-old in the world, and sometimes I find – and she feels I'm cold sometimes, and I am – I know I am, and it bugs me, and I think it's related.

TH: Totally related. You can have a relationship in fantasy, but to have a real relationship and get close to another human being is much more difficult for you.

PT: Right. The doctor said you are someone who helps – and I am sort of a, uh, I guess, I don't know what you call her – a friend, a life coach, from Silva, which is like a spiritual program, but she was very supportive, because what you do it sort of the psychiatrist side of the coin of what the Silva people and the folks I hang out with from a spiritual way – they think there is a continuum from what we are as a child, that we still are –

TH: OK, so are you aware that rather than talking about yourself and what goes on inside of you, you tell me about what other people think – what your wife thinks, your coach thinks, your therapist thinks?

PT: Yeah.

TH: What about you?

PT: I have to. I am desperate.

TH: Actually, you don't have to and it is a choice.

PT: No, no, I really have no choice. I really need help.

TH: Let's look at what is happening here. You have a strong tendency to be dependent – dependent on drugs, pornography, and other people, while taking a passive, subservient position, not just in sex, but generally. You even present yourself here, in a sense, in a passive way – "I have to – I have no choice." This is not true. Of course you have a choice. It is imperative that this is your will to get help, to get to the bottom of this problem, and to get your freedom. Is it your will to free yourself?

PT: You know, I just don't know how to answer that. In some ways, being passive works fine. In other ways, it doesn't. But I know this, that – until I find a will to deal with this situation, it is sort of like – if I was a guy who fell off an ocean liner and got a life preserver, what I'm going to do when I get back to shore, I don't know. But I'm not going to let this take me down.

As in the first case presented here, this man started the session with a long, circuitous monologue that called his cognitive functioning into question. While highly anxious ("like a man walking to the electric chair"), he was tense in his muscles and able to respond meaningfully to inquiry. This suggested that his rambling and evasive responses were primarily due to the habitual use of character defenses including compliance, submissiveness, minimization, idealization, and devaluation. Left in place, these defenses would prevent the development of a genuine alliance and contribute to another treatment failure. In fact, most treatment-resistant patients have character pathology that prevents the kind of emotional engagement required for change to take place. In ISTDP, we work actively with these defenses, and the resistance they create, in an effort to remove these obstacles and forge a therapeutic alliance.

In this case, the patient presented himself in a highly masochistic fashion, stating he was in "hot water" with his wife because he had been a "bad boy." He was attending the consultation in order to please her and do his penance. If the therapist accepted his wife's concern (and that of his other providers), rather than helping him identify his own feelings, wishes, and goals, she would become an unwitting proxy for third parties. In the process, this would reinforce his being in a one-down, beaten position. Such a pattern of interaction would create a collusive alliance between the patient's defenses and the therapist.

This pattern of subservience and compliance with the wishes and demands of others is common in older patients, who often have caretakers involved in their treatment. Until and unless a patient identifies an internal problem for which he seeks help, there is no basis for psychotherapy. Instead, the ISTDP therapist identifies this **transference pattern of behavior** (i.e., the similar ways in which the patient relates both to the therapist and others in his life), challenges the patient to give up destructive ways of relating to himself and others, and encourages him to be open and forthright in order to free himself from suffering.

In the opening sequence of this treatment, the process of identifying defenses and their cost is illustrated. While the patient was highly identified with these character defenses, a focused and persistent approach on their cost yielded benefits. The patient was able to acknowledge his tendency to be subservient and his desire to give it up, in favor of an active approach to tackling his difficulties. Once he declared, "I'm not going to let this take me down," we could begin the work:

TH: So, you have a tendency to take a passive, subservient position with others and to rely on external means of regulating your own internal state – with pornography and drugs. You are also saying that you have a difficulty in the sexual relationship with your wife. What is the nature of the problem?

PT: Anxiety. I make her be the initiator. Once I get started, I'm OK. It's like with public speaking – I get so anxious, but once I get started, I do a pretty good job. I have, I mean, this has been a pattern all my life.

TH: This terrible anxiety. Let's look at that. Are you aware of feeling anxious right now? Where do you feel that tension?

PT: All my, all my voluntary muscles. When I was a better practitioner of relaxation . . .

TH: Well let's just stay in the moment. So, lots of muscle tension, kind of all over, and what else? Anything in your stomach or gut?

PT: No.

This vignette confirms that the patient's anxiety, while quite high, was all bound in muscle tension. As we examined the cost of his externalizing defenses, he became increasingly open about his difficulties. While not overly concerned about his use of pornography, he was quite distressed about his inability to initiate sex with his wife. Now that he had declared a problem he wanted help with, the process could proceed. It is also important to note that his cognitive clarity improved as characterological defenses were given up.

The patient went on to talk about anxiety and his masochistic behavior at work, offering an example of an interaction with a prosecuting attorney who had failed to do an adequate job of representing his client. After suppressing his anger toward opposing counsel for hours, he suddenly blew up, and ended up swearing at him. Then the patient felt guilty, apologized, and volunteered to take on the work the other attorney should have completed! We reviewed this whole pattern of behavior so he could see – and then turn against – his own tendency to suppress anger, explode, apologize, and then do penance.

TH: Do you need some help with this? You say, "Boy, I have trouble dealing with my anger in a healthy, constructive way." You either swallow it and go to this depressive position of "I'm not good" – or, every once in a while, blow up in such a way that you feel guilty, apologize profusely, and then take a beaten position.

PT: Oh yeah. Every time I get angry I end up in one of these, "Oh, no. I have to apologize." As far as experiencing the anger, it's probably what you say – either masking it or going ballistic. I have no notion of anything in the middle.

We agreed that his reliance on pornography was a distraction from his inner life. We also agreed that the chronic use of defenses, including self-attack, self-doubt, passivity, and compliance, exacerbated his symptoms and perpetuated interpersonal dysfunction – in both his personal life and in his work. He took a one-down, beaten position with others, while encouraging others to dominate in all spheres of life.

After obtaining agreement on this formulation of the patient's problems, in the next (second) session, the patient reported a significant breakthrough in his professional life. Following this, he took a big risk in the therapy itself, consolidating this change.

PT: You know, I had a breakthrough the other night. I got on the elevator and there was a guy who I recognized from the newspaper. He had a case that was related to a case I had, and it was just a big thing for me to say, "Are you Steven? My name is Tom. I was wondering, I had a case like yours." It is absolutely something I would not have done years ago.

TH: Wow.

PT: I did it because the curiosity I had about the case overcame my fear.

TH: So, the healthy part of you – the part that wants to connect, that wants to learn from him – was greater than your fear. You actually approached him and initiated a conversation and felt good about yourself instead of avoiding it and feeling bad.

PT: Absolutely. I was really happy that I was able to do that, and kind of proud.

TH: So how do you feel that happy, proud feeling inside right now?

PT: I feel stronger. I feel bigger.

TH: So, it's actually a different feeling inside.

PT: Of yes, it's a physical feeling – instead of being hunched over, I am being erect.

TH: That's also a very interesting word you use that even sexually you have been limp and something has gotten in the way of being strong and erect. So, you can have, for brief moments, the experience of being healthy, strong, initiating contact, feeling good about yourself, and you want that to expand and be your baseline.

PT: Absolutely.

As this change was acknowledged and consolidated, he brought up a topic he would typically avoid – having angry feelings toward me for what he saw as my dismissive attitude regarding his age, expressed in the first session.

PT: You talked about my age and it may seem like if a person reaches the age of 65 and they haven't changed, if you were a betting man, you might bet against them, but –

TH: So, let's look at the feelings that you are having toward me, because you were hearing me challenge you, and maybe even being pessimistic in some way or doubting that could change, had the will to change, were too old, or something like that. Right?

PT: Right. My feeling was, "I don't understand where the doctor is coming from," but I can say, "Screw her. She doesn't understand or let her help."

TH: Those were your thoughts, but what kind of feelings and emotions get triggered toward me? Even though your rational mind can say, "I know she is trying to help me and I'm going to give it a go," doesn't mean you don't have feelings about it. So, what is the feeling toward me?

PT: The first meeting was, "Wow – great. She got me." But then I felt resentment, "Where does she get off?" The comment I felt most angry about was, "You are 65 years old and are still engaging in this activity that you are embarrassed about."

TH: It's great that you can let me know that. How do you experience the anger inside?

PT: I'm not sure what you mean. *(Remember, he had no idea of anything "in between" suppression of anger or acting out.)*

TH: We want to help you create a space to feel this anger without having to do anything about it – not suppressing it and getting anxious, or acting on it and feeling guilty – but letting yourself experience the energy and power that comes with it.

PT: Right.

TH: Do you see what I mean? Tell me what you've got so we can really see if we are partners and in agreement.

PT: I felt comfortable just sharing what the things were that caused me anger and the fact that you didn't react in any way – that's all I need to hear – I feel I'm all right.

TH: You're saying that the fact that you could get in touch with your anger and express it directly, and that I could just listen to you – not get defensive or issue ultimatum – was new. For you to say it. Is that right? It felt new? Like talking to the guy in the elevator. The fact that I listened…

PT: The fact that you listened and didn't take offense, that's all I need. I feel like, what you are doing is – you're saying we are going to make a bond and work on understanding the world together – and understanding *me* together. And it's an extraordinary – unusual and striking and extraordinary – and I didn't expect that. I didn't know you were going to do that. I'm not at all put off by it.

TH: What is the feeling about that?

PT: It's a great thing – that you would try to be my partner in doing this – I'm thrilled.

This interaction constituted a profound **corrective emotional experience**[59] and paved the way for a brief and highly effective treatment. Having asserted himself with a senior colleague and then the therapist, he felt stronger and more confident. No longer anxious, depressed, and slumped over, he felt a sense of healthy pride in his own capacity. This experience enabled him to speak up to his wife for the first time. While he had been more than willing to provide for the family and have her stay home with their son when he was young, his wife never returned to work once the son went to school – even when he left for college. The patient realized he had resented her for spending time and money on tennis, dance lessons, and shopping, while assuming no responsibility for the financial support of the family. Furthermore, he could understand how this buried resentment was manifest in his sexual withholding – and why he got so angry with the other attorney for failing to take responsibility for his client (parallel to his wife and son).

As he allowed himself to experience and express his own wishes, feelings, and desires, his need to avoid them with drugs and pornography disappeared. He gave both up without much struggle. Doing so buoyed his self-confidence even further. He was no longer anxious, self-doubting, and depressed, but calm and self-assured. His passive, subservient manner of relating to others was replaced with collaboration and mutual respect. In addition, once again notice that, in the latter vignettes, his responses appeared tighter and more cogent; his apparent cognitive difficulties resolved with the resolution of these defenses. So, even though "a betting man" – as he put it – might not have given him good odds, he was able to make deep and lasting change in only 10 sessions with the help of an ISTDP therapist. Age, diagnosis, and history are poor predictive variables, but response to intervention in the here-and-now can provide us with the most useful and timely data on the patient's ability to make use of psychotherapy.

Summary/Conclusions

Intensive short-term dynamic psychotherapy is a method of treatment with an accumulating evidence base that it is both clinically effective and cost-effective across a wide range of patients, from those with anxiety and depression, to those with chronic pain, unexplained medical symptoms, character disorders, and conversion. While research is only beginning to examine ISTDP's effectiveness with older adults, both authors have clinical experience in implementing the method with considerable success in this population. These therapeutic results suggest that the widely held belief that older adults are "set in their ways" and cannot make deep and lasting change in their 60s, 70s, and 80s needs to be seriously reexamined. Two cases were presented to illustrate how the use of ISTDP can help assess and treat patients with both multiple symptoms of long-standing and significant character pathology that had prevented the development of a collaborative alliance in previous attempts at treatment. Further research is needed, but this is a promising beginning.

References

1. Yarns BC. Psychotherapy. In: Tampi RR, Tampi DJ, Boyle LL, editors. *Psychiatric disorders late in life: a comprehensive review*. Cham: Springer; 2018. p. 297–306.

2. Dobson KS. *Handbook of cognitive-behavioral therapies*. New York: Guilford Press; 2009.

3. Town JM, Abbass AA, Driessen E, et al. Updating the evidence and recommendations for short-term psychodynamic psychotherapy in the treatment of major depressive disorder in adults: the Canadian Network for Mood and Anxiety Treatments 2016 guidelines. *Canadian J Psychiatry*. 2017;**62**(1):73–74.

4. Leichsenring F, Luyten P, Hilsenroth NJ, et al. Psychodynamic therapy meets evidence-based medicine: a systematic review using updated criteria. *Lancet Psychiatry*. 2015;**2**(7):648–660.

5. Driessen E, Cuijpers P, de Maat SC, et al. The efficacy of short-term psychodynamic psychotherapy for depression: a meta-analysis. *Clin Psychol Rev*. 2010;**30**(1):25–36.

6. Jones EE, Pulos SM. Comparing the process in psychodynamic and cognitive-behavioral therapies. *J Consult Clin Psychol*. 1993;**61**(2):306–316.

7. Society of Clinical Psychology. Short-term psychodynamic therapy for depression. 2018. Retrieved from:

www.div12.org/treatment/short-term-psychodynamic-therapy-for-depression/ (November 13, 2018).

8. Steuer JL, Mintz J, Hammen CL, et al. Cognitive-behavioral and psychodynamic group psychotherapy in treatment of geriatric depression. *J Consult Clin Psychol.* 1984;**52**(2):180.

9. Thompson LW, Gallagher D, Breckenridge JS. Comparative effectiveness of psychotherapies for depressed elders. *J Consult Clin Psychol.* 1987;**55**(3):385.

10. Gallagher-Thompson D, Hanley-Peterson P, Thompson LW. Maintenance of gains versus relapse following brief psychotherapy for depression. *J Consult Clin Psychol.* 1990;**58**(3):371–374.

11. Gallagher-Thompson D, Steffen AM. Comparative effects of cognitive-behavioral and brief psychodynamic psychotherapies for depressed family caregivers. *J Consult Clin Psychol.* 1994;**62**(3):543–549.

12. Cuijpers P, van Straten A, Smit F. Psychological treatment of late-life depression: a meta-analysis of randomized controlled trials. *Int J Geriatr Psychiatry.* 2006;**21**(12):1139–1149.

13. Pinquart M, Duberstein PR, Lyness JM. Effects of psychotherapy and other behavioral interventions on clinically depressed older adults: a meta-analysis. *Aging Ment Health.* 2007;**11**(6):645–657.

14. Huang AX, Delucchi K, Dunn LB, et al. A systematic review and meta-analysis of psychotherapy for late-life depression. *Am J Geriatr Psychiatry.* 2016;**23**(3):261–273.

15. Xie CL, Wang XD, Chen J, et al. A systematic review and meta-analysis of cognitive behavioral and psychodynamic therapy for depression in Parkinson's disease patients. *J Neurol Sci.* 2015;**36**(6):833–843.

16. Lumley MA, Schubiner H. *Emotional exposure therapy for stress reduction: a group-based treatment manual for patients with fibromyalgia and related chronic pain disorders (Version 2).* Detroit, MI: Wayne State University; 2012.

17. Lumley MA, Schubiner H, Lockhart NA, et al. Emotional awareness and expression therapy, cognitive behavioral therapy, and education for fibromyalgia: a cluster-randomized controlled trial. *Pain.* 2017;**158**(12):2354–2363.

18. Burger AJ, Lumley MA, Carty JN, et al. The effects of a novel psychological attribution and emotional awareness and expression therapy for chronic musculoskeletal pain: a preliminary, uncontrolled trial. *J Psychosom Res.* 2016;**81**:1–8.

19. Freud S. *An autobiographical study.* New York: W. W. Norton; 1963/1925.

20. Coughlin Della Selva P. *Intensive short-term dynamic psychotherapy.* London: Karnac; 1994/2006.

21. Freud S. *Inhibitions, anxiety, and symptoms.* Toronto: Longmans, Green; 1936/1926.

22. Davanloo H. *Unlocking the unconscious: selected papers of Habib Davanloo, MD.* New York: Wiley; 1990.

23. Davanloo H. Intensive short-term dynamic psychotherapy: extended major direct access to the unconscious. *European Psychotherapy* 2001;**2**(2):25–70.

24. Bowlby J. *Attachment and loss. Vol. 2: Separation: anxiety and anger.* New York: Basic Books; 1973.

25. Abbass AA. *Reaching through resistance: advanced psychotherapy techniques.* Kansas City, KS: Seven Leaves Press; 2015.

26. Lane RD., Ryan L, Nadel L, et al. Memory reconsolidation, emotional arousal, and the process of change in psychotherapy: new insights from brain science. *Behavioral and Brain Sciences.* 2015;**38**:e1.

27. Ecker UKH, Lewandowsky S, Oberauer K. Removal of information from working memory: a specific updating process. *J Mem Lang.* 2014;**74**:77–90.

28. Shedler J. The efficacy of psychodynamic psychotherapy. *American Psychologist.* 2010;**65**(2):98–109.

29. Abbass AA. Intensive short-term dynamic psychotherapy in a private psychiatric office: clinical and cost effectiveness. *Am J Psychother.* 2002;**56**(2):225–232.

30. Fava GA, Ruini C, Rafanelli C, et al. Six-year outcome of cognitive behavior therapy

for prevention of recurrent depression. *Am J Psychiatry*. 2004;**161**(10):1872–1876.

31. Perlis RH. Cognitive behavioural therapy has short term but not long term benefits in people with residual symptoms of depression. *Journal of Evidence-Based Mental Health*. 2005;**8**(3):75.

32. Menninger K. *Theory of psychoanalytic technique*. New York: Basic Books; 1958.

33. Malan DH. *Individual psychotherapy and the science of psychodynamics*. London: Butterworths; 1979.

34. Ekman P, Friesen WV. Constants across cultures in the face and emotion. *J Pers Soc Psychol*. 1971;**17**(2):124–129.

35. Scherer KR. What are emotions? and how can they be measured? *Social Science Information*. 2005;**44**(4):695–729.

36. Panksepp J. *Affective neuroscience: the foundations of human and animal emotions*. New York: Oxford University Press; 1998.

37. Cramer P. Changes in defence mechanisms during psychoanalysis and psychotherapy: a case study. In: Cohen J, Cohler BJ, editors. *The psychoanalytic study of lives over time: clinical and research perspectives on children who return to treatment in adulthood*. San Diego, CA: Academic Press; 2000.

38. Yarns BC, Wells KB, Fan D, et al. The physical and the emotional: case report, mixed-methods development, and discussion. *Psychodyn Psychiatry*. 2018;**46**(4):553–578.

39. Town JM, Abbass AA, Bernier D. Effectiveness and cost effectiveness of Davanloo's intensive short-term dynamic psychotherapy: does unlocking the unconscious make a difference? *Am J Psychother*. 2013;**67**(1):89–108.

40. Abbass AA, Lovas D, Purdy A. Direct diagnosis and management of emotional factors in chronic headache patients. *Cephalalgia*. 2008;**28**(12):1305–1314.

41. Selye H. A syndrome produced by diverse nocuous agents. *Nature*. 1936;**138**(3479):32.

42. Moran TP, Taylor D, Moser P. Sex moderates the relationship between worry and performance monitoring brain activity in undergraduates. *Int J Psychophysiol*. 2012;**85**(2):188–194.

43. Freud A. *The ego and the mechanisms of defense*. London: Hogarth; 1966/1936.

44. Coughlin P. *Maximizing effectiveness in dynamic psychotherapy*. New York: Routledge; 2017.

45. Davanloo H. *Short-term dynamic psychotherapy*. New York: Jason Aronson; 1980.

46. Davanloo H. Clinical manifestations of superego pathology. Part II: The resistance of the superego and the liberation of the paralyzed ego. *International Journal of Short-Term Psychotherapy*. 1988;**3**(1):1–24.

47. Davanloo H. *Principles and techniques of short-term dynamic psychotherapy*. New York: Spectrum; 1978.

48. Davanloo H. Techniques of short-term dynamic psychotherapy. *Psychiatr Clin North Am*. 1979;**2**:11–21.

49. Abbass AA, Joffres M, Ogrodniczuk J. Intensive short-term dynamic psychotherapy trial therapy: qualitative description and comparison to standard intake assessments. *Ad Hoc Bulletin of Short-Term Dynamic Psychotherapy*. 2009;**13**:6–14.

50. Abbass AA, Kisley S, Town J. Cost-effectiveness of intensive short-term dynamic psychotherapy trial therapy. *Psychother Psychosom*. 2018;**87**(4):255–256.

51. Abbass AA, Town J, Ogrodniczuk J, et al. Intensive short-term dynamic psychotherapy trial therapy: effectiveness and role of "unlocking the unconscious." *The Journal of Nervous and Mental Disease*. 2017;**205**(6):453–457.

52. Aafjes-van Doorn K, Lilliengren P, Cooper A, et al. Patients' affective processes within initial experiential dynamic therapy sessions. *Psychotherapy*. 2017;**54**(2):175.

53. Aafjes-van Doorn K, Macdonald J, Stein M, et al. Experiential dynamic therapy: a

preliminary investigation into the effectiveness and process of the extended initial session. *J Clin Psychol.* 2014;**70** (10):914–923.

54. Gage FH. Neurogenesis in the adult brain. *Journal of Social Neuroscience.* 2002;**22** (3):612–613.

55. Jeste DV, Palmer BW, Rettew DC, et al. Positive psychiatry: its time has come. *J Clin Psychiatry.* 2015;**76**(6):675–683.

56. Pascual-Leone A, Amedi A, Fregni F, et al. The plastic human brain cortex. *Annu Rev Neurosci.* 2005;**28**:377–401.

57. Folstein MF, Folstein SE, McHugh PR. "Mini-mental state." A practical method for grading the cognitive state of patients for the clinician. *Journal of Psychiatry Research.* 1975;**12**(3):189–198.

58. Nasreddine ZS, Phillips NA, Bedirian V, et al. The Montreal Cognitive Assessment, MoCA: a brief screening tool for mild cognitive impairment. *J Am Geriatr Soc.* 2005;**53**(4):695–699.

59. Alexander F, French TM. *Psychoanalytic therapy: principles and application.* New York: Ronald Press; 1946.

Other Therapies: Reminiscence Therapy, Cognitive Behavioral Therapy for Insomnia, and Cognitive Behavioral Therapy for Hoarding Disorder

Renz J. Juaneza, Nery Diaz, and Pallavi Joshi

In preceding chapters, we provided a detailed review of the research and practice of four common, evidence-based psychotherapy approaches for older adults: cognitive behavioral therapy (CBT), problem-solving therapy (PST), interpersonal psychotherapy (IPT), and brief dynamic psychotherapy (BDP). However, many other psychological treatments exist and are of potential interest to the clinician treating older adults. These include all the varieties of cognitive and behavioral therapies; third-wave cognitive behavioral treatments such as acceptance and commitment therapy (ACT) and dialectical behavior therapy (DBT); mindfulness-based approaches such as mindfulness-based stress reduction (MBSR); combined approaches such as those used to treat substance use disorders in the elderly that involve cognitive and behavioral strategies, motivational interviewing, and a 12-step approach; treatments with unique proposed mechanisms, including life review and reminiscence therapies (RT); and treatments for unique conditions such as complicated grief. In addition, numerous other psychosocial/nonpharmacologic treatments do not act directly on psychological processes but are also of interest to the clinician; these include music and art therapy and even garden therapy.

While a detailed review of all these approaches is beyond the scope of this book, the evidence base for many of these treatments is described in other chapters. This chapter provides an overview of three useful approaches chosen by the chapter's authors (RT for depression, CBT for insomnia [CBT-I], and CBT for hoarding disorder [CBT for HD]) based on their experience and expertise and the potential utility of the treatments for clinicians working in both outpatient and inpatient settings.

Reminiscence Therapy for Depression

Introduction

Reminiscence therapy is defined by the American Psychological Association (APA) as "the use of life histories – written, oral, or both – to improve psychological well-being."[1] Similar to its close relative, life review therapy, RT is intended to respect one's life experiences to help maintain good psychiatric/psychological health. Using the aid of prompts such as photos, music, or familiar items from the past, the therapist encourages the patient to talk about memories from earlier in life. Typical topics include family and friendships, failed and successful relationships, achievements and disappointments, and adapting to life changes. Sessions can last from 30–60 minutes and occur at least on a weekly basis.

In the mid-twentieth century, reminiscence had a negative connotation, as it was considered to be a harbinger of psychiatric illness. Talking about distant memories was thought of as "living in the past" and, thus, was considered problematic. However, the emergence of Erik Erikson's stages of psychosocial development helped reshape the potential utility of reminiscence. Erikson's last stage, designated as "late adulthood," introduced the concept of integrity versus despair.[2] During this life stage, it becomes important to reflect on one's life with satisfaction, and, with death occurring at this juncture, the issue of personal integrity becomes prominent. Questions such as, "What do I have to be proud of?" are common in this age group, and this issue is either accepted with satisfaction, or with an air of disappointment and despondence. An individual typically seeks to balance life successes and disappointments in this stage and to philosophically reach an understanding of their meaning to the individual.[3]

By incorporating Erikson's theories, Dr. Robert Butler, a psychiatrist and geriatrician, pioneered the RT movement in 1963. Butler coined the term "life review," which he considered to be a normal part of late life and a way for people to put their lives into perspective. Early reminiscence experiments examined both the cognitive changes and the alterations in personal perceptions that occurred via reminiscing,[4,5] with subsequent research centered on its functions and benefits. By the 1980s, RT was instituted in a group therapy format, resulting in an increase in professionals trained in this therapeutic process.[6]

Types of Reminiscence

The two most prominent and effective types of RT are integrative and instrumental. Integrative RT involves accepting past negative events and resolving them by reconciling the difference between ideals and reality and finding meaning and worth in life.[7] An integrative life review engages older adults to scrutinize their lives and refute negative self-appraisals that cause, or are associated with, depression. It presumes that depressed people tend to ignore positive information and, instead, focus on memories that support their dysfunctional views. Integrative reminiscing spurs patients to recount a comprehensive life story, thus producing a more balanced understanding of their past. Good and bad events are assessed, which in turn illustrates to the patient that negative life experiences are offset by positive occurrences. For example, failure in one's career can be balanced by success in another life domain, such as family life, consequently reducing one's cognitive distortions, such as selective abstraction or catastrophizing.[7] Recalling events in a historical context also allows patients to gain positive perspective of their shortcomings by attributing them to external factors instead of blaming themselves. Watt et al. provide an example of a Great Depression-era teacher who was unable to find a job and ascribed that failure to her substandard teaching skills but was unable to recognize that her unemployment was most likely due to a poor economy.[7] Ultimately, reminiscence creates a realistic and adaptive view of self that incorporates both positive and negative attributes and improves depressive symptoms.

Instrumental RT helps the older adult recall past coping strategies, memories of how difficult situations were resolved, and how aspirations were achieved.[7] This therapy subtype positively affects self-esteem by recalling events where the individual acted effectively to control the environment and resolve stressors. It also helps individuals focus on other goals that are more compatible with their current limitations. Instrumental RT can be especially helpful for the elderly who may not be able to do now what they were once capable of doing.

Reminiscence is also broken down into information, evaluation, and obsessive types.[7] Information reminiscence centers on enjoying retelling stories from the past and is useful for people who lack pleasure in their lives to remind them what they should be happy about.[8] Evaluative reminiscence is considered the main type of RT and involves sharing life memories in a group setting. Obsessive reminiscence is frequently used so one can relinquish lingering guilt.

Evidence for Reminiscence Therapy in Older Adult Depression

Several studies have examined the effects of RT for depressed older adults. A 12-week study found that, by using integrative RT, institutionalized older veterans experienced significant decreases in depressive symptoms with an average improvement of approximately two points on the Geriatric Depression Scale (GDS), Self-Esteem Scale, and Life Satisfaction Index.[9] Another trial showed that integrative and instrumental RT helped participants' long-term affect improve by significantly decreasing depressive symptoms measured by the GDS and Hamilton Rating Depression Scale (HAM-D): 58% of participants achieved symptom remission after 6 weeks of therapy.[7] Reminiscence used as an intervention for a community's older adult suicides showed that after a course of group RT, 97.3% of participants enjoyed the experience of talking, 98.7% enjoyed listening to others, 89.2% felt that the group reminiscence work would help in their daily life, and 92.6% wished to continue in the program.[10] This study also corroborated previously observed effects of increased life satisfaction and self-esteem. The benefits of RT occurred independently of therapy being conducted individually or in groups. The effectiveness of RT was not affected by frequency or duration of therapy, and individuals with higher initial depressive symptoms exhibited a greater rate of improvement of their symptoms. There was an improvement in self-esteem along with a lasting effect across multiple metrics, including wellbeing, ego integrity, and preparation for death.[9]

It should be noted that some depressed individuals naturally reminisce out of boredom, as a way of rehashing bitter memories, or as the end of their life approaches, and may be suitable candidates for formal reminiscence therapy.[10] Additionally, in a bereavement setting, reminiscence may allow people to resolve grief by sharing fond memories of a deceased love one and gaining a sense of peace from their loss.[11]

A few researchers have posited that the positive effects of RT are the result of a patient's ability to cope and deal with new situations effectively through assimilative and accommodative coping.[12] Assimilative coping complements the objective of allowing individuals to pursue their goals regardless of personal limitations and obstacles.[9] Accommodative coping helps individuals adjust their goals to accommodate deficiencies and constraints through revising values and priorities and possibly changing their personal identity.[13] Furthermore, problem- and emotion-focused coping, facilitated by instrumental reminiscence, has been associated with recovery from depression. Problem-focused coping is a goal-oriented, analytical approach to improving symptoms; emotion-focused coping cultivates personal growth through taking personal responsibility for one's own role in creating stress and subsequently looking at the positive aspects of the stress.[7]

Summary of Reminiscence Therapy

Reminiscence therapy is an inexpensive and beneficial approach for helping older adults age successfully and with happiness. Although there are no appreciable adverse effects of this treatment modality, it is important to be cautious during the therapy process as not all memories are pleasant, and depressed patients are susceptible to worsening outcomes if they become overly focused on life's disappointments.[12] Reminiscence appears to provide patients with a sense of life satisfaction and coping skills and ameliorates the symptoms of depression. Despite encouraging results, a caveat is that many studies evaluating reminiscence were only partially controlled and, as such, clinicians should keep their expectations for success realistic and use reminiscence as part of a multi-pronged approach in the treatment of late-life depression. Reminiscence can be categorized under the umbrella of supportive therapy. Available studies clearly demonstrate a significant positive effect of this therapy on mood, self-care, self-esteem, social relationships, ability to communicate, and wellbeing. Individuals also report a more favorable outlook of their past and consequently are more optimistic about their future. Anecdotally, older adults appreciate the opportunity to put their lives into perspective as death approaches, allowing them to feel complete. At the very least, reminiscence can serve as a vehicle for nurturing the therapeutic alliance, in that individuals may be able to verbalize their problems and concerns in a sympathetic environment. At its best, reminiscence can assist individuals in taking inventory of the disappointments and limitations in their lives, establishing realistic goals, improving depressive symptoms, and achieving ego-integrity, fostering a sense of pride in their lives.

Cognitive Behavioral Therapy for Insomnia

Introduction

Gender and age are the most clearly identified demographic risk factors associated with insomnia, with an increased prevalence noted among women and older adults.[14] Insomnia affects 25–45% of adults over the age of 64 years.[15] Other sleep disorders that adversely affect older adults are sleep apnea and periodic limb movement disorders. Sleep apnea affects 24–42% of older adults, and periodic limb movement disorder affects 45% of older adults.[16]

Sleep problems among older adults are associated with illness, chronic diseases, and the medications used to treat those diseases.[17] Quality of sleep also decreases with increased medical comorbidities.[18] Among older adults, CBT-I offers an evidenced-based treatment for insomnia without the negative consequences of sedating medications.

What Is CBT-I?

Cognitive behavioral therapy for insomnia is a nonpharmacological treatment for insomnia that has been shown to be as effective as medication and likely more durable over time.[19] Cognitive behavioral therapy for insomnia is designed to target perpetuating factors that interfere with sleep, such as napping, oversleeping, spending too much time in bed when not asleep, conditioned arousals, and sleep-related stressors. In 2005, the National Institutes of Health (NIH) State of the Science panel supported CBT-I as a first-line therapy for chronic insomnia.[20]

Cognitive behavioral therapy for insomnia is a data-intensive intervention employing a sleep diary and performance graphs to gather sleep parameters that are used in tailoring therapy to the needs of the patient.[21] The goal of treatment is to decrease the amount of time spent awake in bed and increase the efficiency of sleep, that is, the amount of time spent in bed actually sleeping.

Cognitive behavioral therapy for insomnia is generally offered over 4–8 weeks with once-a-week, face-to-face meetings with the therapist.[21] However, some research indicates that CBT-I is also effective in improving sleep in a group therapy format or brief individual telephone consultations.[22]

Why CBT-I for Older Adults?

Studies have shown that 30–60% of older persons have one or more sleep complaints.[23] The cause of sleep problems in the elderly is often multifactorial and is associated with declining health.[17] Insomnia and chronic insomnia are associated with poor quality of life, increased risk for depression, chronic use of hypnotic medication, risk for nursing home placement, and caregiver burnout. Suicidality is one of the most severe consequences of insomnia in late life.[24] A common intervention for insomnia among older adult is the use of sedating medications that have the potential for adverse events such as daytime sedation, falls, and fractures. In contrast, CBT-I provides an evidenced-based treatment for insomnia among older adults without the adverse effects of sedating medications.

Evidence for CBT-I for Older Adults

A systematic review of the management of insomnia disorder for the Agency for Healthcare Research and Quality demonstrated that CBT-I improved sleep efficiency, sleep onset latency (SOL), and wake-time after sleep onset in older adults with insomnia disorder.[25] A pragmatic, two-arm, randomized controlled trial (RCT) to evaluate the clinical effectiveness of sleep hygiene with CBT-I delivered in self-help booklets to 183 adults ages 55–87 reporting insomnia symptoms associated with chronic disease demonstrated that CBT-I improved the quality of sleep, as measured by the Pittsburgh Sleep Quality Index (P < 0.001), Insomnia Severity index (P < .001), and subjective sleep efficiency index (P < 0.01) over the control group without CBT-I. Cognitive behavioral therapy for insomnia was also associated with initially less sleep medication use than the control group.[26] A randomized, controlled, comparative efficacy trial using polysomnography data of 123 community-dwelling older adults with symptoms of chronic and primary insomnia and inflammatory risk demonstrated that CBT-I performed better than Tai Chi in remission of late life clinical insomnia and also showed greater and more sustained improvement in sleep quality, sleep parameters, fatigue and depressive symptoms (all P values < 0.01).[27]

Components of CBT-I

The major components of CBT-I are sleep hygiene, stimulus control, and sleep restriction. Adjunctive or "second line" components include cognitive therapy and relaxation training. Both stimulus control and sleep restriction are helpful for difficulties with sleep onset and sleep maintenance.

Sleep hygiene consists of educating the patient about behaviors that interfere with achieving restful sleep. The usual clinical recommendations are as follows:

- Make sure the bedroom is quiet and dark with a comfortable temperature, mattress, and pillow.
- Avoid heavy alcohol and excessive liquid consumption in the late evening.
- Avoid excess caffeinated beverage consumption, especially after 2 pm.
- Avoid smoking before going to bed or smoking during the night.
- Avoid going to bed hungry.

The concept of stimulus control is based on principles of classical conditioning where a paired stimulus and response is employed with the goal of reestablishing a healthy association of bed (stimulus) with sleep (response).[21] Insomnia becomes a self-exacerbating problem because the individual spends too much time in bed not sleeping and too much time in the bedroom engaged in activities other than sleep. Chronic insomnia triggers feelings of anxiety and frustration, thereby perpetuating a cycle of sleep dysregulation. The instructions for stimulus control include:[21]

- Avoid behaviors such as reading or watching television in the bedroom.
- Use the bed only for sleep or sex; lie in bed intending to go to sleep only when sleepy.
- Get out of bed and leave the bedroom if awake for more than 15 minutes and return to bed only when sleepy – this should be repeated as necessary throughout the night.

Sleep restriction is a controlled form of partial sleep deprivation that limits time in bed. The goal of sleep restriction is to achieve a more consolidated sleep by manipulating a delay in time to bed while maintaining a fixed wake time. This is achieved by establishing a consistent routine for going to bed at night, awakening in the morning, and eliminating naps during the day. At the initiation of the sleep restriction phase of therapy, the patient is instructed to delay the time to bed with the goal of aligning the amount of sleep per night with average total sleep time. Sleep restriction is limited to no less than 4.5 hours of sleep per night. Over the course of the treatment, time to bed is titrated in increments of 15 minutes per week.

Most older adults are good candidates for CBT-I; however, treatment with sleep restriction may exacerbate or precipitate epilepsy, mania, parasomnias, and hypoventilation, and, for these reasons, sleep restriction is contraindicated among individuals with epilepsy, bipolar disorder, parasomnias, and obstructive sleep apnea.

Cognitive interventions are useful for individuals with symptoms perpetuated by negative beliefs surrounding their insomnia and the consequences of poor sleep. As with other cognitive therapies, challenging distorted beliefs can aid in reducing the anxiety about poor sleep.

Relaxation training, including progressive muscle relaxation, diaphragmatic breathing, biofeedback, hypnosis, mindfulness, and aromatherapy are all adjunctive therapies for insomnia that can help the individual enter a calm state of rest.[21]

CBT-I sessions may be summarized as follows:[21]

- Session 1: Clinical evaluation and instruction on the use of a sleep diary to collect sleep data.
- Session 2: Introduction to sleep restriction and stimulus control therapy. A review of sleep data and establishment of sleep restriction parameters.
- Session 3: A review of sleep hygiene, evaluation of the sleep data, and discussion of sleep restriction parameters.

- Sessions 4–7: Evaluation of the sleep data and discussion of sleep restriction parameters.
- Session 8: Education on relapse prevention.

Summary of CBT-I

Cognitive behavioral therapy for insomnia is a non-pharmacological treatment for insomnia that has been found to be as effective as sedating medications and likely more durable over time. The evidence indicating the benefits of CBT-I in helping restore healthy sleep among older adults and the lack of any known adverse effects makes this an excellent treatment modality for older adults with insomnia.

Cognitive Behavioral Therapy for Hoarding Disorder

Introduction

Hoarding behaviors have been described in various disorders, including obsessive compulsive disorder (OCD), schizophrenia, depression, and anorexia nervosa.[28] Hoarding disorder can also occur in the absence of other psychiatric or physical causes and is characterized by urges to save and difficulties discarding items regardless of their inherent value, resulting in accumulations of possessions that clutter the living space and cause functional impairment.[29] The prevalence of hoarding symptoms ranges from 2[30]–5.3%[31] in nongeriatric populations, and is more common, severe, and treatment refractory among older adults.[30–32] Hoarding disorder, compulsive hoarding, and hoarding symptoms can have serious consequences for older adults, such as increased fall risk, fire hazard, poor hygiene, poor nutrition, and social isolation.[28] Negative consequences of hoarding may be particularly salient for older adults.[28,33,34]

Components of CBT for HD

Four etiological factors for hoarding have been suggested: executive functioning deficits related to decision-making, categorization, and organization; excessive emotional attachment to possessions; a tendency toward behavioral avoidance; and faulty beliefs about the nature of possessions.[28,35] A cognitive behavioral model of hoarding behavior proposes a framework based on vulnerability factors such as genetic predisposition, core beliefs about one's identity and adequacy, and cognitive dysfunction.[36] These vulnerability factors contribute to cognitive appraisals about one's possessions, leading to positive and negative emotional responses, resulting in hoarding behaviors. Hoarding behaviors are positively reinforced when individuals feel secure in having objects they feel they need, while negatively reinforced when individuals avoid the unpleasant emotions that accompany discarding or not acquiring desired objects.[36]

Based on this model, CBT for HD has been developed over the past decade.[36] Cognitive behavioral therapy for HD includes motivational interviewing, graded exposure to non-acquiring (gradually building an ability to resist the urge to buy or otherwise acquire items), training in sorting and discarding (practicing effective decision-making), cognitive restructuring (identifying and correcting maladaptive patterns of thinking), and organizational training (practicing appropriate handling and placement of items to be saved in order to reduce clutter in the home).

Cognitive behavioral therapy for HD consists of 26 weekly sessions over approximately six months, with three weekly clinic sessions alternating with a monthly home visit, or a visit to an acquisition site. However, the number of sessions may vary from 15–30 based on severity of hoarding.[36] The approximate structure of the program is:

- Assessment: 2–3 sessions
- Case formulation: 2 sessions
- Practice limiting acquiring: 2 sessions
- Skills training: 2–3 sessions, including organizational and problem-solving skills
- Sorting and discarding practice and cognitive therapy: 15 sessions
- Motivational interviewing to address ambivalence and low insight: parts of several sessions, usually early in treatment
- Relapse prevention: 2 sessions

The flow of treatment varies as therapists alternate their focus between organizing, acquiring, and discarding objects, depending on their clients' immediate goals and motivation, and among cognitive and exposure strategies for clearing clutter.[36]

Evidence for CBT for HD

Outcomes of clinical trials of CBT for HD are generally positive, although many individuals continue to experience some degree of hoarding symptoms and associated impairment at post-treatment.[37] A meta-analysis of 10 trials of CBT for hoarding found that HD symptom severity decreased significantly across all studies.[38] The strongest effects were seen for difficulty discarding, the core behavioral feature of hoarding disorder. Clutter and acquiring showed effects in the moderate range. Female gender, younger age, a greater number of CBT sessions, and a greater number of home visits were associated with better clinical outcomes.[38] The authors suggest that the age-related difference is likely due to differential acquiring outcomes, as compulsive buying behaviors are more common among younger adults than among older adults and were more severe in the data studied. In contrast, a recent meta-analysis of group CBT for HD showed a statistically, but not clinically, significant impact of age on effect size.[39]

Although studies demonstrate the efficacy of CBT for HD in middle-aged adults, with a decrease in hoarding symptoms of 10–21% for group CBT[40–42] and 27–28% for individual CBT,[42,43] there are few RCTs on HD in older adults. Ayers et al. investigated CBT for HD in 12 adults over 65 years.[33] Results demonstrated 14–20% improvement in hoarding severity and depression. However, global improvements, anxiety, disability, and clutter ratings were unchanged at post-treatment and 6-month follow-up.[33] A possible reason that CBT for HD is less effective for older adults is that these patients may have subtle neurocognitive deficits that impair engagement and response to CBT.[44,45]

Summary of CBT for HD

Current evidence for using CBT for HD among older adults shows modest efficacy. Given the serious consequences of hoarding in the geriatric population, further research on the development and testing of an intervention that produces clinically meaningful and lasting change is needed. A potential model may deemphasize cognitive restructuring and focus on specific, concrete between-session assignments.

References

1. Tuleya LG. *Thesaurus of psychological index terms*. Washington, DC: American Psychological Association; 2007.

2. Chiang KJ, Chu H, Chang HJ, et al. The effects of reminiscence therapy on psychological well-being, depression, and loneliness among the institutionalized aged. *Int J Geriatr Psychiatry: A Journal of The Psychiatry of Late Life and Allied Sciences*. 2010;25(4):380–388.

3. Hearn S, Saulnier G, Strayer J, et al. Between integrity and despair: toward construct validation of Erikson's eighth stage. *J Adult Dev*. 2012;19(1): 1–20.

4. Bluck S, Levine LJ. Reminiscence as autobiographical memory: a catalyst for reminiscence theory development. *Ageing Soc*. 1998;18(2):185–208.

5. Lewis CN. Reminiscing and self-concept in old age. *Journal of Gerontology*. 1971;26 (2):240–243.

6. Bornat J. Oral history as a social movement: reminiscence and older people. *Oral History*. 1989;17(2):16–24.

7. Watt LM, Cappeliez P. Integrative and instrumental reminiscence therapies for depression in older adults: intervention strategies and treatment effectiveness. *Aging Ment Health*. 2000;4(2): 166–177.

8. Lo Gerfo M. Three ways of reminiscence in theory and practice. *Int J Aging Hum Dev*. 1981;12(1):39–48.

9. Wu LF. Group integrative reminiscence therapy on self-esteem, life satisfaction and depressive symptoms in institutionalised older veterans. *Journal of Clinical Nursing*. 2011;20(15-16):2195–2203.

10. Fujiwara E, Otsuka K, Sakai A, et al. Usefulness of reminiscence therapy for community mental health. *Psychiatry Clin Neurosci*. 2012;66(1):74–79.

11. Wang JJ. Group reminiscence therapy for cognitive and affective function of demented elderly in Taiwan. *Int J Geriatr Psychiatry: A Journal of The Psychiatry of Late Life and Allied Sciences*. 2007;22 (12):1235–1240.

12. Comana MT, Brown VM, Thomas JD. The effect of reminiscence therapy on family coping. *J Fam Nurs*. 1998;4(2):182–197.

13. Cappeliez P, Robitaille A. Coping mediates the relationships between reminiscence and psychological well-being among older adults. *Aging Ment Health*. 2010;14 (7):807–818.

14. Roth T. Insomnia: definition, prevalence, etiology, and consequences. *J Clin Sleep Med*. 2007;3(5 Suppl):S7–10.

15. Mellinger GD, Balter MB, Uhlenhuth EH. Insomnia and its treatment: prevalence and correlates. *Arch Gen Psychiatry*. 1985;42 (3):225–232.

16. Ancoli-Israel S, Kripke DF, Klauber MR, et al. Sleep-disordered breathing in community-dwelling elderly. *Sleep*. 1991;14 (6):486–495.

17. Ancoli-Israel S, Kripke DF. Prevalent sleep problems in the aged. *Biofeedback Self Regul*. 1991;16(4):349–359.

18. Foley D, Ancoli-Israel S, Britz P, Walsh J. Sleep disturbances and chronic disease in older adults: results of the 2003 National Sleep Foundation Sleep in America Survey. *J Psychosom Res*. 2004;56(5):497–502.

19. Ancoli-Israel S. Sleep and its disorders in aging populations. *Sleep Medicine*. 2009;10 (1 Suppl):S7–11.

20. NIH State-of-the-Science Conference Statement on manifestations and management of chronic insomnia in adults. *NIH Consens State Sci Statements*. 2005;22 (2):1–30.

21. Perlis ML, Jungquist C, Smith MT, Posner D. Cognitive behavioral treatment of insomnia: a session-by-session guide. *Springer Science & Business Media*. 2006 Jun 2;182.

22. Bastien CH, Morin CM, Ouellet MC, Blais FC, Bouchard S. Cognitive-behavioral therapy for insomnia: comparison of individual therapy, group therapy, and telephone consultations. *J Consult Clin Psychol*. 2004;72(4):653–659.

23. McCurry SM, Logsdon RG, Teri L, Vitiello MV. Evidence-based psychological treatments for insomnia in older adults. *Psychol Aging*. 2007;22(1):18–27.

24. Dzierzewski JM, Dautovich ND. Who cares about sleep in older adults? *Clin Gerontol.* 2018;41(2):109–112.

25. Brasure M, MacDonald R, Fuchs E, et al. Management of insomnia disorder. Rockville (MD): Agency for Healthcare Research and Quality (US). 2015. Retrieved from: www.ncbi.nlm.nih.gov/books/NBK343503/

26. Morgan K, Gregory P, Tomeny M, et al. Self-help treatment for insomnia symptoms associated with chronic conditions in older adults: a randomized controlled trial. *Am Geriatr Soc.* 2012;60:1803–1810.

27. Irwin MR, Olmstead R, Carrillo C, et al. Cognitive behavioral therapy vs. Tai Chi for late life insomnia and inflammatory risk: a randomized controlled comparative efficacy trial. *Sleep* 2014;37 (9):1543–1552.

28. Ayers CR, Najmi S, Mayes TL, et al. Hoarding disorder in older adulthood. *Am J Geriatr Psychiatry.* 2015;23(4):416–422.

29. American Psychiatric Association. *Diagnostic and statistical manual of mental disorders* (DSM-5®). Arlington, VA: American Psychiatric Association Publishing; 2013. p. 947.

30. Iervolino AC, Perroud N, Fullana MA, et al. Prevalence and heritability of compulsive hoarding: a twin study. *Am J Psychiatry.* 2009;166(10):1156–1161.

31. Samuels JF, Bienvenu OJ, Grados MA, et al. Prevalence and correlates of hoarding behavior in a community-based sample. *Behaviour Research and Therapy.* 2008;46 (7):836–844.

32. Ayers CR, Saxena S, Golshan S, Wetherell JL. Age at onset and clinical features of late life compulsive hoarding. *Int J Geriatr Psychiatry.* 2010;25(2):142–149.

33. Ayers CR, Wetherell JL, Golshan S, Saxena S. Cognitive-behavioral therapy for geriatric compulsive hoarding. *Behaviour Research and Therapy.* 2011;49 (10):689–694.

34. Diefenbach GJ, DiMauro J, Frost R, Steketee G, Tolin DF. Characteristics of hoarding in older adults. *Am J Geriatr Psychiatry.* 2013;21(10):1043–1047.

35. Frost RO, Hartl TL. A cognitive-behavioral model of compulsive hoarding. *Behaviour Research and Therapy.* 1996;34(4):341–350.

36. Steketee G, Frost R. *Compulsive hoarding and acquiring: therapist guide.* 2nd ed. New York: Oxford University Press; 2014.

37. Tolin DF. Understanding and treating hoarding: a biopsychosocial perspective. *J Clin Psychol.* 2011;67(5):517–526.

38. Tolin DF, Frost RO, Steketee G, Muroff J. Cognitive behavioral therapy for hoarding disorder: a meta-analysis. *Depress Anxiety.* 2015;32(3):158–166.

39. Bodryzlova Y, Audet JS, Bergeron K, O'Connor K. Group cognitive-behavioural therapy for hoarding disorder: systematic review and meta-analysis. *Health Soc Care Community.* 2018;25(5):701–9.

40. Muroff J, Steketee G, Himle J, Frost R. Delivery of internet treatment for compulsive hoarding (D.I.T.C.H.). *Behaviour Research and Therapy.* 2010;48 (1):79–85.

41. Muroff J, Steketee G, Rasmussen J, et al. Group cognitive and behavioral treatment for compulsive hoarding: a preliminary trial. *Depress Anxiety.* 2009;26(7):634–640.

42. Steketee G, Frost RO, Tolin DF, Rasmussen J, Brown TA. Waitlist-controlled trial of cognitive behavior therapy for hoarding disorder. *Depress Anxiety.* 2010;27 (5):476–484.

43. Tolin DF, Frost RO, Steketee G. An open trial of cognitive-behavioral therapy for compulsive hoarding. *Behaviour Research and Therapy.* 2007;45(7):1461–1470.

44. Mantella RC, Butters MA, Dew MA, et al. Cognitive impairment in late-life generalized anxiety disorder. *Am J Geriatr Psychiatry.* 2007;15(8):673–679.

45. Caudle DD, Senior AC, Wetherell JL, et al. Cognitive errors, symptom severity, and response to cognitive behavior therapy in older adults with generalized anxiety disorder. *Am J Geriatr Psychiatry.* 2007;15 (8):680–689.

Psychotherapy and Cognitive Disorders

Cynthia A. Kraus-Schuman, Melissa L. Sanchez,
Karen M. Benson, and Ali Abbas Asghar-Ali

Approximately 50 million people worldwide have dementia, and nearly 10 million new cases of dementia are diagnosed every year.[1] Major neurocognitive disorder (dementia) is characterized by significant cognitive decline in one or more cognitive domains (complex attention, executive function, learning and memory, language, perceptual-motor, or social cognition), and these cognitive deficits interfere with independence in everyday activities.[2] Mild Neurocognitive Disorder (mild cognitive impairment [MCI]) is characterized by modest cognitive decline in one or more cognitive domains without interference with independence in everyday activities.[2]

Psychosocial interventions for neuropsychiatric symptoms of dementia (e.g., depression, anxiety, aggression) may be preferable to medications because of risks often present in older adults with dementia related to increased adverse drug reactions, preexisting medical conditions, and complicated medication regimens. In addition, given the mixed evidence base for psychotropic use for neuropsychiatric symptoms in dementia, the use of psychotropic medication is recommended only after attempting behavioral and environmental modifications and appropriate medical interventions.[3] Exceptions to this recommendation include the presence of aggression, causing risk to self or others; major depression with or without suicidal ideation; or psychosis, causing harm or with significant risk of causing harm.[3] Despite their promise and recommendations for their use, nonpharmacological therapies for individuals with dementia have a limited research base and warrant continued development and evaluation. An overview of the most researched interventions for individuals with cognitive impairment and appropriate modifications to psychotherapy for individuals with cognitive difficulties will be described in this chapter.

Assessment

Assessments are often helpful prior to starting any intervention in order to determine the need for the intervention and the preferences and abilities of the individual. Among individuals with dementia, clarifying any overlap of medical symptoms, medication side effects, and the presence of symptoms of anxiety and depression that may contribute to cognitive decline and distress is essential.[4] Memory and communication difficulties can pose challenges to information gathering, hence the value of prior records and collateral information from family and friends. Cognitive and functional assessments (for example, independent activities of daily living and activities of daily living assessments) of the individual with dementia are essential for treatment planning, including adapting the treatment to best suit the abilities of the individual.[4] Psychologists, neuropsychologists, and occupational therapists are just a few of the clinicians who can contribute to these assessments.

Brief standard cognitive examinations like the Mini-Mental State Examination,[5] and the Montreal Cognitive Assessment (MoCA)[6] can be used as part of the evaluation of a person with cognitive changes. Psychiatric symptomatology can be measured using assessments specifically designed for individuals with dementia. In such assessments, the information provided by the individual with dementia is combined with collateral information from other sources, such as caregivers and a review of the records.

The next sections highlight the most common symptoms targeted in interventions for individuals with dementia.

Anxiety and depression. Anxiety and depressive symptoms are common among individuals with dementia or mild cognitive impairment. Anxiety symptom prevalence ranges from 8–71%[7] in individuals with dementia and from 10–74% in individuals with mild cognitive impairment.[8] Prevalence of depressive symptoms in those with dementia ranges from 10–62%[9] and from 36[10]–63%[11] in individuals with mild cognitive impairment.

Anxiety and depression symptoms in individuals with dementia have been linked to decreased quality of life, increased behavioral problems, limitations in activities of daily living,[12, 13] and risk of nursing-home placement.[14,15] Many older adults with dementia may have distressing psychiatric symptoms without meeting the criteria for a specific syndrome. Accordingly, when working with such individuals, clinicians should target the symptoms causing distress. Standardized assessment scales such as the Rating Anxiety in Dementia scale[16] and the Cornell Scale for Depression in Dementia[17] can help with case conceptualization and symptom monitoring.

Lack of pleasurable activities and an increase in aversive events due to decreased functioning can lead to depression in individuals with dementia.[18] Additionally, a focus on limitations and awareness of cognitive difficulties can foster depressed mood and anxiety.[18] Therapists may consider these elements in case conceptualization and treatment planning, including psychotherapy.

Pain. Older adults with dementia have a significantly higher prevalence of bothersome pain (63.5%) and activity-limiting pain (43.3%) than individuals without dementia (54.5% and 27.2%, respectively).[19] Pain is often undertreated and unrecognized in individuals with dementia because of their difficulties with communication and clinicians' challenges to interpret behavioral patterns such as pacing, vocalizations, and aggression; these behaviors could be in response to pain or other causes of distress.[20]

Modifications of Psychotherapy for Individuals with Mild-to-Moderate Cognitive Difficulties

Interventions are discussed using the terms *clinician* and *provider*. *Clinician* is used to refer to the professional taking the lead in developing the intervention and skill use with the individual. *Provider* is used to refer to other professionals and staff members (such as physicians, nursing staff, nurse aides, caregivers, etc.) who support the intervention and individual's use of skills.

The cognitive limitations that affect an individual's ability to remember, comprehend, and apply new skills present challenges for psychotherapy.[21] Modifications can be made to the content, structure, and learning strategies used in session to help adapt interventions to the needs of the individual.[21] Sessions, generally, will be briefer (30–40 minutes) to adjust for fatigue and limitations in attention. A caregiver, provider, or supportive other can participate when the individual needs assistance with practice and skill use outside the session. The complexity of skills should match the abilities and preferences of the individual and the availability of a coach to assist with skill practice and use. In general, behaviorally focused interventions are preferred for people with greater cognitive impairment.

The clinician needs to assess the individual's and coach's understandings of the skill during session. This assessment could involve having the individual and/or coach describe the skill and/or observing the individual and coach practice a skill together.[21] Using a concrete homework plan and written homework directions can also guide continued practice. Organization and memory aides, such as skill reminder cards to keep in a wallet or post in a prominent place (e.g., bedside or kitchen table) and a therapy binder for summary handouts, can also enhance the individual's use of the skill.[21-23] If attention or language/reading is a particular weakness, consider using pictures versus printed words for handouts and reminder cards. Incorporating technology (e.g., email or cell phone reminders) should also be explored to facilitate skill learning and use, both for the individual with dementia and supportive others. Access to therapy can be improved by identifying the different settings in which therapy can be provided, such as in the home, over the telephone, or through videoconferencing, and by nontraditional clinicians and providers (e.g., skill practice facilitated by caregivers). Clinicians might consider training nursing home staff or other caregivers on coaching skills outside of session.

Cognitive Behavioral Therapy

Anxiety and depression. There is growing research support for cognitive behavioral therapy (CBT)-based interventions for individuals with dementia and anxiety or depression. Case studies[4, 21, 24-26] and randomized controlled trials (RCTs)[22, 27] support CBT-based interventions targeting anxiety in individuals with dementia. Also, behaviorally based interventions have led to improvements in depression for both patients and caregivers.[28]

Cognitive behavioral therapy trials [22, 27] have used flexible, skill unit-based interventions that could be tailored to preferences and needs of the individual. Spector and colleagues[27] trained patient-caregiver dyads in CBT skill use—psychoeducation about CBT and anxiety in dementia, self-monitoring, identifying and practicing strategies for feeling safe, identifying and challenging unhelpful cognitions, behavioral experiments, calming thoughts and addressing realistic negative automatic thoughts for anxiety in dementia. Optional modules (interpersonal difficulties and unhelpful rules for living) were also made available. Pairs participated in up to 10 weekly, hour-long sessions. At 15 weeks and at 6 months, differences in anxiety between CBT and treatment as usual (TAU) approached significance, with the CBT group having lower ratings of anxiety. Although the CBT intervention targeted anxiety, the more significant finding was in depression ratings. At 15 weeks and at 6 months, the CBT group continued to have significantly lower depression ratings than the TAU group.

The Peaceful Mind program combined telephone sessions and home visits to teach individuals with dementia and their coaches (adults who spent at least eight hours per week with patients) simplified CBT skills (self-monitoring, deep breathing, behavioral activation, coping self-statements and sleep hygiene).[22] Cognitive behavioral therapy sessions were provided weekly to individuals with dementia and coach pairs (30–60 minutes) for 12 weeks, followed by 8 telephone "booster sessions" over 3 months. After initial skills training sessions, individuals with dementia reported higher quality of life; clinicians rated individuals with dementia as less anxious than individuals receiving usual care. Coaches reported less distress related to the individual's anxiety. This study, along with other skill-based interventions, has not shown positive effects to be sustained for more than six months. This may be because of the progressive nature of dementia. Continued provider facilitation may be needed to help adapt skills to the individual's cognitive and functional changes and changes in the individual-with-dementia–coach relationship, including the addition of clinicians caring for the individual or a change in the individual's living circumstances, e.g., moving to a nursing home. Larger studies of longer duration that evaluate the effectiveness of CBT for anxiety and depression in dementia are needed to validate these findings.

Pain. Cognitive behavioral therapy is the best-documented psychological intervention for pain in individuals with mild-to-moderate dementia.[29] Geriatric multimodal CBT incorporates individuals' values to develop motivational themes for family, clinicians and providers to use in promoting behavioral change.[30] In addition to consulting with individuals and their families, other clinicians, such as medical, nursing, rehabilitation, and dietician staff, can contribute to the prioritization of treatment goals, which can include improved pain tolerance, increased involvement in pleasurable activity, behavioral pain management (e.g., ice and heat, distraction), reductions in negative moods, and decreased frequency of inappropriate behaviors.[30] Sessions can be conducted with family and other care facility providers present, such as certified nursing assistants, who then participate in skill implementation outside session. Eight sessions of Geriatric Multimodal CBT resulted in significant reductions in pain, depression, activity interference due to pain, and emotional distress due to pain, and significant increases in most activities of daily living in nursing-home residents with mild-to-moderate cognitive impairment.[31] Individuals also had significant reductions in intensity, frequency, and duration of their behavioral disturbances.[31]

Cognitive Behavioral Therapy Modifications

Elements of CBT can be simplified to make the skills more accessible to individuals with cognitive difficulties. For example, simplified breathing techniques can be used by both individuals and their supportive others as an introductory, portable, calming skill. Clinicians or caregivers can help the individual with self-monitoring to provide targets for intervention and a means to assess symptom improvement. The clinician can simplify cognitive restructuring by suggesting "calming thoughts" to decrease distress rather than relying solely on the individual independently developing alternative thoughts.[21–23] Elements of behavioral activation can be collaboratively developed (clinician, therapist, individual, supportive others, etc.) to promote an increase in pleasurable events, possibly tailored from prior activities to suit the individual's current needs and abilities. The basic CBT session structure (homework review, skill acquisition or review, new homework) can remain the same.[22,23,32]

Modifications – such as working collaboratively with the individual, family and providers; developing interdisciplinary structured treatment plans; and addressing problems significant to the individual – can contribute to favourable outcomes in pain management for individuals with dementia.[31] This collaborative intervention framework inclusive of the individual's values is a beneficial approach in geriatric interventions, including other forms of psychotherapy.

Problem-Solving Interventions

Problem-solving therapy (PST) is based on a social problem-solving model and considers psychological symptoms as person–environment mismatch. Therefore, a specific problem impacts an individual in different ways at different times due to changes in the individual's physical abilities, cognitive functioning, and environmental conditions.[33] The focus of PST is initiation of effective problem-solving processes across a wide range of challenging situations to alter maladaptive coping, reduce negative emotional responses, and improve self-efficacy.[34] Problem-solving therapists directly teach effective problem-solving skills via a multistep approach that includes problem definition, goal setting, generation and evaluation of alternative solutions, solution selection and planning, and evaluation of solution efficacy.[35]

Although only a few studies examined the use of PST in older adults with cognitive difficulties,[34,36,37] mounting evidence indicates this modality's utility for reducing depressive symptoms,[38] suicidal ideation (SI),[39] and disability[36] in this population. Trials of PST with older adults show acceptability of the therapy when delivered in multiple treatment settings to meet the needs of older individuals and their caregivers, including primary care settings;[40] via telephone, internet, or videophone;[41,42] and inhome settings.[41]

Alexopoulos and colleagues[36] compared PST modified for executive dysfunction to supportive therapy (ST) in older adults with major depression and executive dysfunction. Outcomes indicated greater reductions in disability and depression for PST (versus ST) during treatment and following treatment conclusion.[36] In addition, PST showed greater impact than ST among individuals with more cognitive impairment.[36] Modifications to traditional PST include a directive approach, with increased structure to support initiation of action planning, sequencing, and conclusion of action following goal achievement. Emphasis on positive problem orientation, or an individual's appraisal of problems, emotional responses to problems, and beliefs about ability to engage successfully in problem-solving, often leads to a focus on less complex problems and goals during the learning process to foster this positive problem orientation.[43,44]

Among a sample of depressed, older individuals with cognitive impairment and associated disability, modified problem adaptation therapy (PATH) was compared to ST, with significantly greater reduction in depressive symptoms observed in participants administered inhome PATH compared to those offered inhome treatment with supportive therapy.[42] Furthermore, participants provided PATH (versus ST) were more likely to exhibit remission or partial remission at all time points of the treatment.[42] The PATH protocol emphasized emotion regulation (reductions in negative emotional experience and increases in positive emotions), and clinicians facilitated the identification of situations that triggered negative emotions or dampened positive emotions.[42] Then, compensatory strategies promoted the participation in pleasant activities that allowed participants to avoid situations that triggered negative emotions, often with caregiver participation to facilitate environmental modifications.

Problem-Solving Modifications

Problem-solving therapy allows adaptations based on ability status, cognitive strengths and limitations, environmental challenges, and availability of caregiver support for the intervention, and appears well suited for older adults with cognitive impairment. Adjustments to PST that may be helpful for older adults with CI include a focus on smaller, achievable goals at the outset; use of handouts to increase focus and provide structure; and focus on emotion regulation. In addition, collaborative discussion to identify when caregiver participation may be beneficial (e.g., instances when a problem situation cannot be solved and emotion-focused coping is appropriate) can enable environmental modifications, support avoidance of negatively charged situations, and facilitate behavioral activation.[42]

Mindfulness-Based Interventions

Mindfulness-based interventions involve the individual becoming aware of physical feelings, thoughts and emotions in the present moment without judgment. Mindfulness-based stress reduction (MBSR) is an intervention that incorporates meditation, yoga, mindful breathing and informal mindfulness techniques.[45] Mindfulness-based stress reduction has been shown to be effective in reducing anxiety and depression and in improving cognition in healthy older adults.[46] Over the past decade, interventions extending MBSR to older adults with CI have increased, although the research base remains small.

A small number of MBSR studies suggest benefits for older adults with MCI, including significant improvements in cognitive function and trait mindfulness,[47] and a trend toward improvement in resilience, hopefulness, and perceived stress.[48]

There is emerging research on the use of MBSR in individuals with dementia. In an RCT pilot study, adults with mild-to-moderate dementia in care homes participated in either hour-long, twice-weekly group MBSR sessions for five weeks or treatment as usual.[49] Care home staff were oriented to mindfulness skills to increase with practice their ability to support participants. Mindfulness-based stress reduction modifications included increased emphasis on modelling techniques and more frequent guidance during meditation practices. Group size was reduced to allow more time for individual instruction, and simplified skills were emphasized, such as mindful breathing, attention training, and sensory elements. A significant improvement in quality of life was noted in the MBSR group. Sessions with mindful breathing were the most highly rated. Other skills rated highly by participants were body-based practices (mindful movement and body scan) and mindful listening. A floor effect may account for the absence of significant changes in depression and anxiety in these small studies.

In long-term residential settings, residents, including those with moderate-to-severe dementia, participated in a comparison study between a mindfulness program Present in Now (PIN) and a cognitive therapeutic activities program.[50] Present in Now included attention skill exercises, body-awareness activities, and compassion meditation. During PIN and for 20 minutes afterwards, participants had decreases in agitation, anger, and anxiety/fear ratings, and an increase in pleasurable affect ratings. The cognitive therapeutic activity participants did not show significant improvements in affect.

Mindfulness-based stress reduction may also benefit both individuals with dementia and caregivers. When MBSR was offered to individuals with progressive cognitive decline–caregiver pairs, both reported an increase in quality of life and a decrease in depressive symptoms.[51] The need remains for more research with larger sample sizes and RCTs in order to examine MBSR for individuals with cognitive impairments.

Mindfulness-Based Intervention Modifications

Adaptations to mindfulness interventions that should be considered among older adults with cognitive impairment include highlighting focused attention training; mindful breathing; sensory skills, which focus on one sense at a time (sight, touch, smell, and sound); and increased use of modeling in session.[49] A mindful warm-up activity may help increase engagement and orient participants to the intervention.[49] Frequent guidance during meditation can help address confusion and monitor distress and physical discomfort.[49] If yoga is incorporated, modifications to reduce risk of injury to older adults may be needed.[52]

For individuals with more significant cognitive impairment, incorporating sensory experiences such as aromatherapy (scent), calming and/or preferred types of music (sound), family pictures (sight), favorite movies (sight), or textured blankets (touch) can be pleasurable and help ease distress.[53] For individuals who wander, allowances should be made for them to walk about the room or leave and return later. With a mindful approach that accepts all that the present moment brings, clinicians can consider incorporating individuals' agitation into group by joining with them to use mindful walking.[53] While walking with them, the clinician or provider can encourage individuals to be aware of their bodily sensations of walking and the sights, sounds, and smells around them.

Reminiscence Therapy for Dementia

Reminiscence therapy (RT) involves discussion (in group or individual sessions) of past experiences with aides to trigger memories, such as photographs, music and items from the past. Examples of reminiscence interventions include the life review/life-story book approach (focusing on sessions producing a life-story book), the specific reminiscence approach (also producing a life-story book but focused on specific elements of an individual's life, rather than an entire history), and the general individual reminiscence approach (each session focused on a life phase with memory objects related to each period of an individual's life).[54]

Trials of life review in session to produce a life-story book with memory triggers had outcomes suggesting psychosocial benefits for individuals with dementia.[55,56] A reminiscence intervention was associated with improvements in caregiver strain, staff knowledge regarding residents, and behavioral functioning.[57] Reminiscence therapy using a lifebook was found to lessen depression symptoms in individuals with mild-to-moderate dementia when compared to TAU matched pairs.[58]

The research base for RT is small, with mostly descriptive and observational studies. Despite the minimal research base, the popularity of RT with clinicians and participants warrants its further development and assessment.[59] Any clinician or provider can consider incorporating discussion of pleasurable aspects or events of an individual's life during visits, even if the visit is not psychotherapy focused. Having individuals focus on discussing something pleasant such as a positive memory or aspect of their life that they are proud of can help reduce anxiety and/or boost mood, and this pleasant discussion can assist in rapport building between the clinician and individual.

Treating Behavioral and Psychological Symptoms in Moderate-to-Severe Dementia

As dementia progresses, challenging behaviors can emerge. Individuals with advanced dementia almost universally have at least one behavioral and psychological symptom of dementia (BPSD),[15] which can include hitting, screaming, pacing, wandering, agitation, and decreased inactivity.[60] Clinicians might consider using assessments such as the Neuropsychiatric Inventory[61] to assess behaviors related to dementia. Because of multiple factors contributing to BPSD, including environmental and interpersonal elements, CBT conceptualizations can guide the development of interventions for individuals with dementia and for their caregivers.

Conceptual models directing the treatment of challenging behaviors include the Cohen-Mansfield "unmet needs" perspective, the environmental vulnerability paradigm, and the learning/behavior paradigm.[62,63] The unmet needs paradigm focuses on precipitants of BPSD, such as unmet emotional (i.e., sadness, fear, etc.), social (i.e., being lonely), and physical needs (pain, hunger, etc.). In the environmental vulnerability paradigm, individuals may need assistance in changing and/or coping with environmental stimuli, such as decreasing noise, to decrease behavioral and psychological symptoms of dementia. The learning/behavior paradigm focuses on teaching clinicians, providers, and families to understand problematic behaviors by examining patterns of antecedents, behaviors, and consequences. These models can be used collaboratively to understand challenging behaviors and develop interventions.[63]

A number of nonpharmacological interventions show promise for decreasing BPSD (e.g., environmental interventions, structured activities, staff training, behavior-focused interventions, and sensory or social contact).[63] However, most studies have small numbers of participants or are case studies. The implementation of nonpharmacological approaches for managing challenging dementia-related behaviors in long-term care settings has been limited for numerous reasons, including staff training needs and organizational implementation requirements, such as leadership buy-in.[64]

Summary

The evidence base for psychosocial interventions for older adults with cognitive impairments is growing. In general, clinicians should consider using simplified skills and shortened sessions, increasing the number and frequency of sessions, reducing group size, and providing more guidance during skill instruction and practice when working with individuals with cognitive impairments. More research is needed to develop clinical recommendations for specific techniques as well as to understand the elements of successful interventions (timing, duration, etc.). Finally, there is a need for development of training and support for caregivers to use these interventions.

References

1. World Health Organization. *Dementia*. Retrieved from: www.who.int/news-room/fact-sheets/detail/dementia (October 18, 2018).

2. American Psychiatric Association. *Diagnostic and statistical manual of mental disorders*. 5th ed. Arlington, VA: American Psychiatric Publishing; 2013.

3. Kales HC, Gitlin LN, Lyketsos CG. Management of neuropsychiatric symptoms of dementia in clinical settings: recommendations from a multidisciplinary expert panel. *J Am Geriatr Soc.* 2014;62:762–769.

4. Rehm IC, Stargatt J, Willison AT, Reser MP, Bhar SS. Cognitive behavioral therapy for older adults with anxiety and cognitive impairment: Adaptations and illustrative case study. *J Cogn Psychother.* 2017;31 (1):72–88.

5. Folstein MF, Folstein SE, McHugh PR. "Mini-mental state." A practical method for grading the cognitive state of patients

for the clinician. *J Psychiatr Res.* 1975;**12**:189–198.

6. Nasreddine ZS, Phillips NA, Bédirian V, et al. The Montreal Cognitive Assessment, MoCA: a brief screening tool for mild cognitive impairment. *J Am Geriatr Soc.* 2005;**53**(4):695–699.

7. Seignourel PJ, Kunik ME, Snow L, Wilson N, Stanley M. Anxiety in dementia: a critical review. *Clin Psychol Rev.* 2008;**28**:1071–1082.

8. O. L. Lopez, I. T. Becker, R. A. Sweet. Non-cognitive symptoms in mild cognitive impairment subjects. *Neurocase.* 2005;**11**:65–71.

9. Enache D, Winblad B, Aarsland D. Depression in dementia: epidemiology, mechanisms, and treatment. *Curr Opin Psychiatry.* 2011;**24**(6):461–472.

10. Palmer K, Berger AK, Monastero R, Winblad B, Bäckman L, Fratiglioni L. Predictors of progression from mild cognitive impairment to Alzheimer disease. *Neurology.* 2007;**68**: 1596–1602.

11. Solfrizzi V, D'Introno A, Colacicco AM, et al. Incident occurrence of depressive symptoms among patients with mild cognitive impairment–the Italian Longitudinal Study on Aging. *Dement Geriatr Cogn Disord.* 2007;**24**:55–64.

12. Neville C, Teri L. Anxiety, anxiety symptoms, and associations among older people with dementia in assisted-living facilities. *Int J Ment Health Nurs.* 2011;**20**:195–201.

13. Schultz SK, Hoth A, Buckwalter K. Anxiety and impaired social function in the elderly. *Ann Clin Psychiatry.* 2004;**16**(1):47–51.

14. Gibbons LE, Teri L, Logsdon R, et al. Anxiety symptoms as predictors of nursing home placement in patients with Alzheimer's disease. *J Clin Geropsychol.* 2002;**8**(4):335–342.

15. CG Lyketsos, MC Carillo, JM Ryan, et al. Neuropsychiatric symptoms in Alzheimer's disease. *Alzheimers Dement.* 2011;**7**:532–539. doi:10.1016/j. jalz.2011.05.2410

16. Shankar KK, Walker M, Frost D, et al. The development of a valid and reliable scale for rating anxiety in dementia (RAID). *Aging Ment Health.* 1999;**3**:39–49.

17. Alexopoulos GS, Abrams RC, Young RC, Shamoian CA. Cornell scale for depression in dementia. *Biol Psychiatry.* 1998;**23**:271–84.

18. Teri L, Gallagher-Thompson D. Cognitive-behavioral interventions for treatment of depression in Alzheimer's patients. *Gerontologist.* 1991;**31**(2):413–416.

19. Hunt LJ, Covinsky KE, Yaffe K, et al. Pain in community-dwelling older adults with dementia: results from the National Health and Aging Trends Study. *J Am Geriatr Soc.* 2015;**63**:1503–1511.

20. Husebo BS, Achterberg WP, Lobbezoo F, et al. Pain in patients with dementia: A review of pain assessment and treatment challenges. *Norsk Epidemiologi.* 2012;**22**(2):243–251.

21. Kraus CA, Seignourel P, Balasubramanyam V, et al. Cognitive behavioral treatment for anxiety in patients with dementia: two case studies. *J Psychiatr Pract.* 2008;**14**:186–192.

22. Stanley MA, Calleo J, Bush AL, et al. The peaceful mind program: a pilot test of a cognitive-behavioral therapy-based intervention for anxious patients with dementia. *Am J Geriatr Psychiatry.* 2013;**21**(7):696–708. doi: 10.1016/j. jagp.2013.01.007

23. Paukert AL, Kraus-Schuman C, Wilson N, et al. *The peaceful mind manual:* a protocol for treating anxiety in persons with dementia. *Behav Modif.* 2013;**37**(5):631–664.

24. Kipling T, Bailey M, Charlesworth G. The feasibility of a cognitive behavioural therapy group for men with mild/moderate cognitive impairment. *Behav Cogn Psychother.* 1999;**27**(02):189–193.

25. Koder DA. Treatment of anxiety in the cognitively impaired elderly: Can cognitive-behavior therapy help? *Int Psychogeriatr.* 1998;**10**(02):173–182.

26. García-Alberca JM. Cognitive-behavioral treatment for depressed patients with

Alzheimer's disease. An open trial. *Arch Gerontol Geriatr.* 2017;**71**:1–8.

27. Spector A, Charlesworth G, King M, et al. Cognitive-behavioral therapy for anxiety in dementia: pilot randomized controlled trial. *Br Jf Psychiatry.* 2015;**206**:509–516. doi:10.1192/bjp.bp.113.140087

28. Teri L, Logsdon RG, Uomoto J, McCurry SM. Behavioral treatment of depression in dementia: a controlled clinical trial. *J Gerontol.* 1997;**52B**(4):159–166.

29. Snow AL, Jacobs ML. Pain in persons with dementia and communication impairment. In: Pachana NA, Laidlaw K, editors. *The Oxford handbook of clinical geropsychology.* New York: Oxford University Press; 2014. p. 876–908.

30. Clifford PA, Cipher DJ, Roper KD, Snow AL, Molinari V. Cognitive-behavioral interventions for long-term care residents with physical and cognitive disabilities. In: Gallagher-Thompson D, Steffen AM, Thompson LW, editors. *Handbook of behavioral and cognitive therapies with older adults.* New York: Springer; 2008. p. 76–101.

31. Cipher DJ, Clifford PA, Roper KD. The effectiveness of geropsychological treatment in improving pain, depression, behavioral disturbances, functional disability, and health care utilization in long-term care. *Clin Gerontol.* 2007;**30**(3):23–40.

32. Charlesworth G, Sadek S, Schepers A, Spector A. Cognitive behavior therapy for anxiety in people with dementia: a clinician guideline for a person-centered approach. *Behav Modif.* 2015;**39**(3):390–412.

33. Nezu AM, Nezu CM. *Problem-solving training home based primary care treatment manual.* Washington, DC: Veteran's Health Administration; 2015.

34. Kiosses DN, Ravdin LD, Gross JJ, et al. Problem adaptation therapy for older adults with major depression and cognitive impairment: A randomized clinical trial. *JAMA Psychia.* 2015;**72**(1):22–30.

35. Renn BN, Areán PA. Psychosocial treatment options for major depressive disorder in older adults. *Curr Treat Options Psychiatry.* 2017;**4**(1):1–12.

36. Alexopoulos G, Raue P, Kiosses D, et al. Problem-solving therapy and supportive therapy in older adults with major depression and executive dysfunction effect on disability. *Arch Gen Psychiatry.* 2011;**68**(1):33–41.

37. Alexopoulos G, Raue P, Arean P. Problem-solving therapy versus supportive therapy in geriatric major depression with executive dysfunction. *Am J Geriat Psychiatry.* 2003;**11**(1):46–52.

38. Arean PA, Raue P, Mackin RS, et al. Problem-solving therapy and supportive therapy in older adults with major depression and executive dysfunction. *Am J Psychiatry.* 2010;**167**(11):1391–1398.

39. Gustavson KA, Alexopoulos GS, Niu GC, et al. Problem-solving therapy reduces suicidal ideation in depressed older adults with executive dysfunction. *Am J Geriatr Psychiatry.* 2016;**24**(1):11–17.

40. Arean P, Hegel M, Vannoy S, et al. Effectiveness of problem-solving therapy for older, primary care patients with depression: results from the IMPACT project. *Gerontologist.* 2008;**48**(3):311–323.

41. Choi NG, Marti CN, Bruce ML, et al. Six-month postintervention depression and disability outcomes of in-home telehealth problem-solving therapy for depressed, low-income homebound older adults. *Depress Anxiety.* 2014;**31**:653–661.

42. Kiosses DN, Alexopoulos GS. Problem-solving therapy in the elderly. *Curr Treat Options Psychiatry.* 2014;**1**(1):15–26.

43. Gellis ZD, Nezu AM. Integrated depression care for homebound medically ill older adults: using evidence-based problem-solving therapy. In: Sorocco KH, Lauderdale, S, editors. *Cognitive behavior therapy with older adults: innovations across care settings.* New York: Springer; 2011. p. 391–420.

44. Arean PA, Raue P, Mackin RS, et al. Problem-solving therapy and supportive therapy in older adults with major depression and executive dysfunction. *Am J Psychiatry.* 2010;**167**(11):1391–1398.

45. Kabat-Zinn J. *Full catastrophe living: using the wisdom of your body and mind to face stress, pain, and illness.* New York: Dell; 1990.

46. Serpa JG, Taylor SL, Tillisch K. Mindfulness-based stress reduction (MBSR) reduces anxiety, depression, and suicidal ideation in veterans. *Med Care.* 2014;52:S19–S24.

47. Wong WP, Coles J, Chambers R, et al. The effects of mindfulness on older adults with mild cognitive impairment. *J Alzheimers Dis Rep.* 2017;1(1):181–193.

48. Wells RE, Kerr CE, Wolkin J. Meditation for adults with mild cognitive impairment: a pilot randomized trial. *J Am Geriat Soc.* 2013;61(4):642–645.

49. Churcher Clarke A, Chan JMY, Stott J, et al. An adapted mindfulness intervention for people with dementia in care homes: feasibility pilot study. *Int J Geriatr Psychiatry.* 2017;32(12):e123–e131.

50. Kovach CR, Evans C, Sattell L, et al. Feasibility and pilot testing of a mindfulness intervention for frail older adults and individuals with dementia. *Res Gerontol Nurs.* 2018;11(3):137–150.

51. Paller KA, Creery JD, Florczak SM, et al. Benefits of mindfulness training for patients with progressive cognitive decline and their caregivers. *Am J Alzheimers Dis Other Dement.* 2014;30(3):257–267.

52. Wetherell JL, Hershey T, Hickman S, et al. Mindfulness-based stress reduction for older adults with stress disorders and neurocognitive difficulties. *J Clin Psychiatry.* 2017;78(7):e734–e743.

53. McBee L. Mindfulness practice with the frail elderly and their caregivers. *Top Geriatr Rehabil.* 2003;19(4):257–264.

54. Subramanian P, Woods B. The impact of individual reminiscence therapy for people with dementia: systematic review. *Expert Rev Neurother.* 2012;12(5):545–555.

55. Haight BK, Gibson F, Michel Y. The Northern Ireland life review/life storybook project for people with dementia. *Alzheimers Dement.* 2006;2:56–58.

56. Subramanian P, Woods B, Whitaker C. Life review and life story books for people with mild to moderate dementia: a randomized controlled trial. *Aging Ment Health.* 2014;18(3):363–375.

57. Thorgrimsen L, Schweitzer P, Orrell M. Evaluating reminiscence for people with dementia: a pilot study. *Arts Psychother.* 2002;29(2):93–97.

58. Bohlken J, Weber SA, Siebert A, et al. Reminiscence therapy for depression in dementia. *GeroPsych.* 2017;30:145–151. doi: 10.1024/1662-9647/a000175

59. Woods B, Spector AE, Jones CA, Orrell M, Davies SP. Reminiscence therapy for dementia. *Cochrane Database Syst Rev.* 2009;2:1–36.

60. Moniz Cook E, De Vugt M, Verhey F, James I. Functional analysis-based interventions for challenging behavior in dementia. *Cochrane Database Syst Rev.* 2009;3:1–7.

61. Cummings JL, Mega MS, Gray K, et al. The neuropsychiatric inventory: comprehensive assessment of psychopathology in dementia. *Neurology.* 1994;44:2308–2314.

62. Cohen-Mansfield J. Nonpharmacologic interventions for inappropriate behaviors in dementia: a review, summary, and critique. *Am J Geriatr Psychiatry.* 2001;9(4):361–381.

63. McGee JS, Bratkovich KL. Assessment and cognitive-behaviorally oriented interventions for older adults with dementia. In: Sorocco KH, Lauderdale S, editors). *Cognitive behavior therapy with older adults: innovations across settings.* New York: Springer; 2011. p. 219–261.

64. Karel MJ, Teri L, McConnell E, Visnic S, Karlin BE. Effectiveness of expanded implementation of STAR-VA for managing dementia-related behaviors among veterans. *Gerontologist.* 2015;56(1):126–134. doi:10.1093/geront/gnv068

10 Combining Psychotherapy and Medications for Late-Life Psychiatric Disorders

Meera Balasubramaniam, Deepti Anbarasan, and Paul Campion

Introduction

The field of psychiatry has witnessed a multitude of changes over the years, including the furthering of psychopharmacology, integration with the neurosciences, the growing emphasis on evidence-based medicine, a move toward deinstitutionalization, and the advent of managed care. An unexpected and perhaps unintended component of this changing landscape has been the demarcation between psychopharmacology and psychotherapy as independent entities in psychiatric care. Treatment visits are frequently labeled as "therapy" and "medication management" visits, while psychiatrists have come to be known as "psychopharmacologists" or "prescribers" in some settings. The many changes notwithstanding, treatment resistance remains a problem we often contend with in managing patients with mental illnesses. The Sequenced Treatment Alternatives to Relieve Depression (STAR*D) demonstrated that only a fraction of patients achieved full symptom remission. While systematic and sequential trials of anti-depressants certainly helped some patients with treatment-resistant depression, the odds of full recovery progressively diminished with every additional step.[1] Adverse childhood experiences, personality disorders, comorbid substance use, and limited social support are often associated with treatment resistance.[2,3] The ongoing problem of treatment resistance has given impetus to the development of newer medications and the evolution of many forms of neurostimulation, all of which have yielded positive results. In contrast, our understanding of why the above-mentioned factors contribute to treatment ineffectiveness remains limited.

This environment of treatment resistance has brought back the focus on psychotherapy. We ask if combining the two entities would cut through treatment resistance and result in better outcomes. In this chapter, we will first argue that psychotherapy and psychopharmacology are not as independent as they have come to be seen. We will use a case to elucidate that effective treatment entails an ongoing application of psychological concepts and psychotherapeutic skills, even in the context of "medication management" visits. Aspects unique to the treatment of older adults will be highlighted. Following that, we will present a review of the literature on combining psychotherapy with medications for the treatment of late-life psychiatric disorders.

Psychological Considerations in Pharmacotherapy

The Case of Mr. M

Mr. M is a 72-year-old man, a retired university professor. He presents to Dr. S, a woman in her early 30s, for the treatment of depression. He suffered a stroke two years ago, following which he has been experiencing weakness and stiffness on his left side. He has been living by himself following the death of his wife five years ago. Since the stroke, his two adult children, who live in different cities, have been visiting him very frequently to help. He is the eldest of four siblings. His father died by suicide when he was 10 years old, following which his mother started drinking heavily. Mr. M recalls being "the able one" in his family who helped educate his younger siblings. His youngest brother died by suicide 10 years ago, after years of "treatment that failed him". Mr. M enjoyed several supportive friendships, although he has distanced himself from his friends since the stroke. His former psychiatrist prescribed fluox- etine for him over a year ago, without any improvement in his symptoms. Mr. M presents as pleasant, affable, and well-spoken. He describes feeling depressed for over a year. He attributes the stroke to "making me this person I don't recognize" and describes themes of helplessness. He laments that, formerly an avid tennis player, he now ambulates with a cane. He speaks with fondness and pride about his years as a professor, and often remarks that he is a shadow of his former self.

Their sessions consist of providing Mr. M with a space in which he feels understood and supported, one in which he can outline his losses, examine the conflict between a sense of control and the need for assistance, as well as discuss what being depressed and receiving treatment means to him. After careful consideration of Mr. M's presentation, Dr. S prescribes him mirtazapine at their second session. She meets with him every two weeks for the first three months of treatment and on a monthly basis after that. She also refers him to a local senior center. Mr. S experiences significant improvement in his mood and overall outlook. He starts socializing with friends once again. By the end of six months, Mr. M's depression has remitted.

The above vignette illustrates an effective treatment, one in which the patient progressed from a scenario of nonresponse to treatment, to one of complete illness remission. One can attribute the change to alpha-2 presynaptic blockade brought about by mirtazapine, some- thing that could not be achieved with fluoxetine. But one cannot overlook other distinguish- ing aspects of this treatment process. These include the therapeutic alliance and the development of a thoughtful biopsychosocial formulation. We cannot conclusively deter- mine the relative contributions of the two factors to symptom remission. But there is evidence to show that synthesis of biological and psychological insights enhances the overall treatment outcome.[4,5] In the following section, we will use the case of Mr. M as a template to highlight salient nonpharmacological aspects to be considered in order to achieve effective outcomes in pharmacotherapy.

Understanding the Meaning of Illness and Treatment

A purely biological framework provides the prescribing clinician with information about the patient's illness course, severity, and treatment history. But it does not adequately provide a glimpse into the factors that determine individuals' sense of self, their personality and relational characteristics, or their capacity for change. Older adults frequently face losses in the form of the death of loved ones and the loss of youth and vitality. They also fear losing independence. Many individuals struggle to maintain their self-esteem in the context of these biopsychosocial losses. Illness states such as depression are often viewed by older adults as a personal flaw, representing their inability to adequately cope with life circum- stances. It is noteworthy that Dr. S prescribed mirtazapine at the second visit and continued to meet her patient every two weeks during the initial phase of treatment. This time investment and her emphasis on understanding Mr. M as an individual allowed him to discuss the loss of his wife and friends, to mourn the loss of his healthy former self, and to explore the ambivalence he experienced at receiving assistance from his children. He also shared the feelings of sadness, humiliation, and fear he often experienced. He was able to do so in an environment where he could feel validated and supported. Dr. S was able to help Mr. M disentangle his own depression as distinct from the long-held resentment toward his father and brother, who had died by suicide. This was a crucial first step toward his recovery.

A solely biological explanation of mental illness carries the risk of promoting a view of oneself as victim to a chemical imbalance. Applying a psychosocial frame and emphasizing one's internal resources helps preserve personal agency in one's recovery.[6] By suggesting that Mr. M actively participate in the activities at his senior center, Dr. S emphasized that he had an active role in his recovery. Depending upon the patient and treatment context, this can take the shape of behavioral activation, encouragement to engage in pleasurable activities, or maintaining a mood diary, thus cutting across different types of psychotherapies. Treatment expectation is another dynamic and modifiable factor that impacts the outcome. The correlation between treatment expectations and the response to antidepressants has been demonstrated.[7] Individuals like Mr. M who have experienced childhood neglect are likely to approach treatment and professional caregivers with caution. Mintz and Flynn recommend asking specific questions and setting a space to address ambivalence, one in which patients can openly discuss how likely they are to stop a medication if they were to either experience side effects or not experience appreciable improvement.[6]

Applying Interpersonal Processes to Pharmacotherapy

While it is known that medication resistance is frequently encountered among individuals with personality disorders, we seldom focus on how disordered object relations negatively influence the response to medications.[8] Older adults present unique transferential issues. Grunes described the phenomenon of reverse transference in the relationship between elderly patients and young clinicians, one in which the clinician is viewed as a child of the patient.[9] Some young clinicians feel overwhelmed while dealing with medical problems, losses, and the fear of death that older patients experience.[10] In the absence of adequate appreciation for this dynamic, the anxiety may be translated into the urge on the part of clinicians to increase medication doses or to prescribe complex regimens beyond what is clinically warranted. Attachment patterns, which play out in the treatment alliance between the patient and the clinician, equally determine the relationship between patients and their medications.[6] Secure attachments are positively associated with response to antidepressants, while insecure–anxious attachments are linked to greater incidence of side effects and premature discontinuation.[6,11]

By offering Mr. M a safe and trusting relationship, Dr. S was able to understand the negative mental association he had with fluoxetine, a medication that had been prescribed to his brother, who had died of suicide. She provided him with a positive pharmacotherapeutic relationship and elicited Mr. M's preference in treatment before prescribing mirtazapine.

Additionally, clinicians must incorporate the dynamic understanding of a patient into their prescribing techniques and titration schedules. It is imperative to follow a "start low, go slow" strategy for ambivalent patients who express apprehensions about side effects of medications. On the other hand, in the case of a patient who is skeptical about treatment effectiveness but indifferent to side effects, the clinician may consider adopting a somewhat more aggressive dosing strategy.[6]

The vignette described thus illustrates the importance of consistently assimilating psychological factors into pharmacotherapy. We believe this integrated approach will add value to all clinical settings. Even in split treatment, it is possible to effortlessly blend psychotherapy and pharmacotherapy with collaborative working relationships and regular communication between clinicians.

Review of the Literature

The National Institute for Health and Clinical Excellence has recommended that all patients with severe, treatment-resistant or recurrent depression should be treated with a combination of antidepressant medications and individual cognitive behavioral therapy (CBT).[12] To date, limited literature exists on the efficacy of combined treatment with both psychotherapy and medications in geriatric patients with psychiatric conditions.

Combined Therapy in Depression

Several studies have evaluated the efficacy of combining antidepressants and psychotherapy, most often interpersonal psychotherapy (IPT) or cognitive behavioral therapy, in the treatment for late-life depression.

Reynolds and colleagues performed the first randomized controlled study of maintenance pharmacotherapy and psychotherapy in late-life depression.[13] The authors sought to determine the efficacy of maintenance nortriptyline and IPT in preventing recurrence of major depressive episodes in patients older than 59 years. They noted that IPT, when combined with nortriptyline, was an effective acute treatment in older adults with recurrent major depression.

Additionally, combined treatment was seen to be superior to IPT alone (P = 0.003) and showed a trend to superior efficacy compared to medication alone (P = 0.06) in terms of preventing recurrence, especially during the first year of treatment and in patients aged 70 years and older. The authors noted that combined treatment helped prevent or delay recurrence of mood symptoms and opined that this was the optimal clinical strategy for elderly patients with major depression. They identified that this effect may be attributable to some clinical characteristics common to elderly patients, including high levels of medical comorbidities; impaired sleep quality; and frequently occurring psychosocial stressors like role transitions, interpersonal conflict, and bereavement.

Lenze and colleagues examined whether maintenance treatment of late-life depression with combined nortriptyline and IPT would be more likely to help patients maintain social adjustment than either modality alone.[14] Forty-nine subjects who were 60 years and older and had diagnoses of recurrent, nonpsychotic major depression completed the study. Social adjustment was measured using the Social Adjustment Scale. The mean scores on the scale improved in the combined treatment group, but declined in the monotherapy groups. The authors concluded that subjects who received combination therapy better maintained improvements in social adjustment and enhanced the length and quality of recovery. They also specifically noted that they saw the greatest impact in the domain of interpersonal conflict, which was suggestive of the specific effects of IPT combined with medication in terms of maintaining better social functioning in patients with late-life depression.

Thompson and colleagues performed a randomized controlled trial (RCT) with 102 subjects in which they evaluated the efficacy of desipramine alone, CBT alone, or combination therapy in treatment of depression in major depressive disorder (MDD) in late life.[15] Both the combined group and CBT-alone group had similar rates of improvement; however, when stratified by depression severity, the more severely depressed patients (based on a standardized depression scale) receiving combined treatment showed greater improvement than either modality alone. Combination therapy resulted in greater improvement in depression than desipramine.

Hollon et al. performed a literature review to compare the relative efficacy of medications or psychotherapy alone or in combination for treatment of depression.[16] The authors found that medications were effective for rapid, robust treatment while continued but lost their efficacy when discontinued. Ongoing IPT and CBT also appeared to reduce risk of relapse, though they noted that CBT appeared to have an enduring effect that reduced risk after termination. The authors concluded that combined treatment with medication and psychotherapy retained the benefits of each modality and likely enhanced the probability of response over monotherapy in chronic depression.

Combined Therapy in Anxiety

The literature supports the use of selective serotonin reuptake inhibitors as a first-line pharmacological treatment for generalized anxiety disorders (GADs) in the geriatric population. However, anxiety and pathological worry in the elderly may be more resistant to treatment with medications or CBT, when compared to anxiety in younger adults.

In a RCT, Schuurmans and colleagues evaluated the effectiveness of sertraline in management of anxiety disorders in 84 individuals over the age of 60.[17] The subjects were assigned to 1 of 3 arms: 15 sessions of CBT, pharmacological treatment with sertraline for 3 months, or a waitlist control group. They noted that both CBT and sertraline led to improvement in anxiety, worry, and depressive symptoms at 3-month follow-up, but that sertraline was most efficacious for worry symptoms. The combined mean effect size for all 3 outcomes (anxiety, worry, depressive symptoms) of sertraline (mean d = 1.02) was much higher at 3-month follow-up when compared to CBT (mean d = 0.35). The authors opined that further study was merited to assess the utility of using antidepressants to treat anxiety in older adults. In a follow-up study, the authors contacted the subjects 1 year after completion of the trial to examine long-term outcomes.[18] Again, sertraline showed a greater reduction of symptoms than CBT on anxiety and worry ratings with a higher effect size for sertraline (mean d = 0.92) than CBT (mean d = 0.35) at the time of 1-year follow-up. The authors suggested that maintenance treatment with sertraline might be more beneficial in the long run for the treatment of late-life anxiety than a standard CBT program.

Wetherell and colleagues performed an open label pilot study to evaluate the efficacy of augmenting medication with modular cognitive behavioral therapy (mCBT).[19] Modular cognitive behavioral therapy differs from fixed-session standardized CBT models, as modular designs allow clinicians to tailor treatment toward the individual's specific needs and circumstances. The study included 12 subjects who were at least 60 years old and met *Diagnostic and Statistical Manual of Mental Disorders* (DSM-IV) criteria for a principal diagnosis of GAD of at least moderate intensity. In the first phase of the study, subjects received 12 weeks of open-label escitalopram, followed by 16 weeks of escitalopram augmented with mCBT, and then a 28-week period during which medications were tapered off. During the first phase of treatment, the mean Hamilton Anxiety Rating Scale (HAM-A) score decreased from 23.3 to 13.0 and the mean Penn State Worry Questionnaire (PSWQ) score decreased from 55.5 to 49.8. Following the second phase, the mean HAM-A score decreased to 8.2 and the PSWQ decreased to 40.9. After discontinuation of the medication, at the end of the maintenance phase, the mean HAM-A score was 13.3. Specific PSWQ scores were not available, but only 2 patients remained in remission at the end of the maintenance phase based on PSWQ criteria (remission indicated by score < 40). Three patients relapsed during this phase and were placed back on medications. The authors concluded that the planned sequential treatment approach of an antidepressant augmented by mCBT was an effective strategy. The study highlighted the finding that anxiety symptoms, as measured by the HAM-A, appeared to respond better to medications, whereas worry, as measured by the PSWQ, seemed to respond better to psychotherapy. The authors also commented on how open, consistent communication between pharmacotherapists and psychotherapists did not interfere with treatment and that patients were appreciative of combination therapy.

Wetherell and colleagues performed a follow-up investigation in which they evaluated whether sequenced treatment, combining pharmacotherapy and mCBT, boosts response and prevents relapse in older adults with generalized anxiety disorder.[20] In this study, 73 subjects who were at least 60 years of age were first given 12 weeks of open-label escitalopram and were then assigned to one of four groups: (1) 16 weeks of escitalopram plus mCBT, followed by 28 weeks of maintenance escitalopram, (2) 44 weeks of escitalopram alone, (3) 16 weeks of escitalopram plus mCBT followed by 28 weeks of pill placebo, and (4) 16 weeks of escitalopram followed by placebo. The response rate did not differ significantly between the escitalopram-plus-mCBT group and the escitalopram-only group, although the former group exhibited greater improvements in pathological worry, as measured by the Penn State Worry Questionnaire. No significant difference was noted in the HAM-A scores between these groups. Subjects assigned to escitalopram in the maintenance phase had significantly lower relapse rates when compared to those receiving placebo, regardless of prior mCBT exposure. For subjects on placebo in the maintenance phase, those who received mCBT had lower rates of relapse compared to those who did not receive modular cognitive behavioral therapy. The findings indicated that medication followed by augmentation with mCBT led to improvement in worry severity, though not anxiety symptoms, in older adults with generalized anxiety disorder. They also highlighted that both maintenance medication and mCBT were beneficial for relapse prevention.

In a meta-analysis of 32 studies focused on anxiety disorders in older adults by Pinquart and Duberstein, pharmacotherapy was felt to be more effective than behavioral interventions in reducing anxiety symptoms, with an effect size of 1.76 for pharmacotherapy and an effect size of 0.81 for behavioral interventions.[21] The authors noted that these effect sizes were similar or even larger than those reported in similar studies in younger patients, negating the concept that older patients benefit less from treatment options than younger patients.

Conclusion

This chapter has described the complex interplay between psychopharamacology and psychotherapy for elderly patients. Even with the current arsenal of pharmacological interventions, a significant number of patients suffer from treatment-resistant symptoms.

Psychiatrists may be hopeful about the additional efficacy expected from relatively new modalities of treatment, from medication classes such as N-methyl-D-aspartate (NMDA) antagonists to methods of neurostimulation. However, there remains a significant component of treatment resistance that is conferred from less "biological" sources, commonly thought to include trauma history, maladaptive behavior, and social isolation. For this aspect of treatment, psychotherapy is an essential intervention. Psychotherapy may allow patients to closely explore these factors in a way that is impossible during routine medication management visits.

The clinical vignette highlighted the role of supportive psychotherapy in conjunction with thoughtful medication management, resulting in remission of depressive symptoms. Psychological factors affecting elderly patients are too complex to be reduced to stereotypes. However, one may construct a framework of the "general concerns" of elderly patients, which must be refined over the course of treatment.

Erik Erikson formulated the last stage of life as the "fruit" of all the stages that preceded it. In the healthy personality, this stage becomes a time when one may consider the summation of an entire life. One may conclude with a sense of overall satisfaction or, as Erikson described it, "integrity." However, if one cannot derive a sense of integrity, Erikson postulated that one may experience despair. Despair may surface as misanthropy or displeasure with particular people or institutions, and is ultimately a projection of one's own self-disgust.[22]

Common transferential and countertransferential issues regarding the care of elderly patients can include a reverse transference and the therapist's feeling of helplessness or being overwhelmed. Other common stressors that may be considered in the psychological formation can include: deceased friends and family, isolation, and loss of independence (whether physical or financial).

Later in this chapter, the literature was reviewed regarding combined medication and psychotherapy in elderly patients. Overall, the literature is limited. However, existing studies suggest that the efficacy of combined medication management and psychotherapy for depression is superior to either modality alone. The acute response phase as well as the durability of effect for combined treatment may also be superior to either treatment alone. Regarding anxiety in elderly patients, the literature suggests that medication management may be more effective than behavioral interventions, although there is some evidence that worry symptoms (as measured by PSWQ) may respond better to cognitive behavioral therapy. More research is needed to determine which psychotherapeutic intervention is best suited to a particular symptom subtype (such as anxiety or worry) of an anxiety disorder.

References

1. Warden D, Rush AJ, Trivedi MH, Fava M, Wisniewski SR. The STAR*D project results: a comprehensive review of findings. *Current Psychiatry Reports*. 2007 Dec 1;9 (6):449–459.

2. Drapeau M, Perry JC. Childhood trauma and adult interpersonal functioning: a study using the core conflictual relationship theme method (CCRT). *Child Abuse & Neglect*. 2004 Oct 1;28 (10):1049–1066.

3. Zisook S, Johnson GR, Tal I, et al. General predictors and moderators of depression remission: a VAST-D report. *Am J Psychiatry*. 2019 Apr 5; appiajp201818091079.

4. Gabbard GO. Psychodynamic psychiatry in the" decade of the brain." *Am J Psychiatry*. 1992 Aug;149(8):991–998.

5. Vlastelica M. Psychodynamic approach as a creative factor in psychopharmacotherapy. *Psychiatria Danubina*. 2013 Sep 17;25(3):0–319.

6. Mintz DL, Flynn DF. How (not what) to prescribe: nonpharmacologic aspects of psychopharmacology. *Psychiatric Clinics*. 2012 Mar 1;35(1):143–163.

7. Krell HV, Leuchter AF, Morgan M, Cook IA, Abrams M. Subject expectations of treatment effectiveness and outcome of treatment with an experimental antidepressant. *J Clin Psychiatry*. 2004 Sep;65(9):1174–1179.

8. Mintz D, Belnap B. A view from Riggs: treatment resistance and patient authority – III. What is psychodynamic psychopharmacology? An approach to pharmacologic treatment resistance. *J Am Acad Psychoanal Dyn Psychiatry*. 2006 Dec;34(4):581–601.

9. Leigh R, Varghese F. Psychodynamic psychotherapy with the elderly. *J Psychiatr Pract*. 2001 Jul 1;7(4):229–237.

10. Atiq R. Common themes and issues in geriatric psychotherapy. *Psychiatry (Edgmont)*. 2006 Jun;3(6):53.

11. Comninos A, Grenyer BF. The influence of interpersonal factors on the speed of recovery from major depression. *Psychother Res*. 2007 Mar 1;17(2):230–239.

12. National Institute for Health and Clinical Excellence. *Depression: management of depression in primary and secondary care.* NICE; 2004.

13. Reynolds CF 3rd, Frank E, Perel JM, et al. Nortriptyline and interpersonal psychotherapy as maintenance therapies for recurrent major depression: a randomized controlled trial in patients older than 59 years. *JAMA*. 1999b;281:39–45.

14. Lenze EJ, Dew MA, Mazumdar S, et al. Combined pharmacotherapy and psychotherapy as maintenance treatment for late-life depression: effects on social adjustment. *Am J Psychiatry*. 2002 Mar;159(3):466–468.

15. Thompson LW, Coon DW, Gallagher-Thompson D, Sommer BR, Koin D. Comparison of desipramine and cognitive/behavioral therapy in the treatment of elderly outpatients with mild-to-moderate depression. *Am J Geriatr Psychiatry*. 2001;9:225–240.

16. Hollon SD, Jarrett RB, Nierenberg AA, et al. Psychotherapy and medication in the treatment of adult and geriatric depression: which monotherapy or combined treatment? *J Clin Psychiatry*. 2005 Apr;66(4):455–468.

17. Schuurmans J, Comijs H, Emmelkamp PM, et al. A randomized, controlled trial of the effectiveness of cognitive-behavioral therapy and sertraline versus a waitlist control group for anxiety disorders in older adults. *Am J Geriatr Psychiatry*. 2006;14:255–263.

18. Schuurmans J, Comijs H, Emmelkamp PM, et al. Long-term effectiveness and prediction of treatment outcome in cognitive behavioral therapy and sertraline for late-life anxiety disorders. *Int Psychogeriatr*. 2009;21:1148–1159.

19. Wetherell JL, Stoddard JA, White KS, et al. Augmenting antidepressant medication with modular CBT for geriatric generalized anxiety disorder: a pilot study. *Int J Geriatr Psychiatry*. 2011 Aug;26(8):869–875.

20. Wetherell JL, Petkus AJ, White KS, et al. Antidepressant medication augmented with cognitive-behavioral therapy for generalized anxiety disorder in older adults. *Am J Psychiatry*. 2013 Jul;170(7):782–789.

21. Pinquart M, Duberstein PR. Treatment of anxiety disorders in older adults: a meta-analytic comparison of behavioral and pharmacological interventions. *Am J Geriatr Psychiatry*. 2007 Aug;15(8):639–651.

22. Erikson E. *Identity and the Life Cycle.* New York: W.W. Norton; 1980.

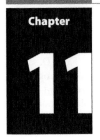

Chapter

Psychotherapy with Diverse Adults in Later Life

Sarah A. Nguyen, Philip Blumenshine, and Boski Patel

Introduction

Psychiatrists working with older adults encounter diagnostic and therapeutic challenges that are often more complex than those in young adult and middle-aged patients.[1] The approach to psychotherapy for older adults should account for the patient's cultural background and identity. According to the US Census Bureau, nonwhites are expected to account for more than half the U.S. population by 2050.[2] The concept of "Culturally Diverse Populations" now includes groups defined by age, gender, gender identity, language, country of origin and acculturation, sexual orientation, socioeconomic status, religion/spirituality, and geographic location.[3] With the growing aging population, it is increasingly important to understand specific challenges that these minority groups may face in older age, and the implications of these challenges in a psychotherapeutic context.

Since the 1980s, growing attention has been paid to the role of race and ethnicity in psychiatric treatment, but specific evidence-based treatments and guidelines for psychotherapy in racially and ethnically diverse older populations remain limited. Clinicians working with older adults may benefit from developing cultural formulations referencing the cultural formulation appendix of the DSM-5.[4] For older racial and ethnic minorities, additional psychiatric considerations include the cultural context for the presenting problem, differing religious/spiritual beliefs, and various acculturation considerations for immigrant minorities. Prior research suggests that older adults have a harder time acculturating to new environments due to language barriers, deep roots in their respective home countries, and lack of readily available social groups.[5-7]

Additionally, older adults can also be characterized by cohort, which is defined as a group of individuals who experience the same event at the same time. Conceptually, certain abilities, beliefs, attitudes, and personality dimensions remain stable with age and can characterize and distinguish cohorts born earlier and later.[8] Although cohort differences are not developmental, understanding older adults is as much about understanding people who matured in a specific era as it is about understanding the physiological aging process. In this chapter, we will provide an overview of psychotherapeutic challenges unique to diverse populations among older adults, while acknowledging that substantial research remains to be done. We will also highlight specific cohort concerns relevant to older adults currently in or about to enter psychotherapy treatment.

Racially and Ethnically Diverse Older Adults

Because the origins of conventional psychotherapy are based on the cultural context dominant in North America and Western Europe,[9] the values and worldviews of ethnic and racial minority groups may be culturally incongruent with conventional psychotherapy modalities. Although "race" refers to a person's physical characteristics (such as bone structure and skin, hair, or eye color), and "ethnicity" refers to cultural factors (including nationality, regional culture, ancestry, and language), the two will be used interchangeably throughout this section, as studies overall are limited in examining ethnic and racial differences. It has been suggested that racially and ethnically matched dyads avoid cross-group stereotypes and improve both the therapeutic alliance and treatment effectiveness since shared ethnicity has usually been viewed as a proxy for shared background experiences.[10] Although studies show patients prefer being matched to a mental health treatment provider of the same race/ethnicity,[10,11] concrete markers of treatment success, such as dropout rates and measures of symptom reduction, show inconsistent and, at most, very small effects.[12] Particularly in the diagnosis of depression, race concordance may be associated with decreased frequency of diagnosis.[13]

What appears more effective is adapting psychotherapy in ethnically and racially appropriate ways. The American Psychiatric Association (APA) developed the Cultural Formulation Interview (CFI) as a structured interview tool to assess presenting problems based on the patient's cultural definition and perception, as well as incorporating cultural factors related to the patient's psychosocial environment and cultural elements affecting the provider-patient relationship.[4] Just as the CFI adapted the standard, ethnocentric psychiatric interview to culturally diverse groups, therapists can also adapt psychotherapy to take a patient's cultural values, contexts, and worldview into account. Although most psychotherapy research develops and tests evidence-based treatments among European Americans, more recent literature indicates the effectiveness of culturally adapted psychotherapy, which is defined as the systematic modification of protocols based on culture and context to align more with a patient's values, contexts, and worldviews.[14,15] Consideration of cultural factors in the emergence of a problem, help-seeking and service utilization, factors that may affect accurate diagnosis, therapeutic and treatment issues, and posttreatment adjustment must all be considered in the psychotherapeutic framework.[16,17] Patients can then feel safe enough to elaborate on culturally appropriate feelings in therapy.[10,18]

Latinos compromise a diverse ethnic and racial mix of peoples with different languages, traditions, and beliefs. Like that for Asian and African Americans, data on psychotherapeutic modalities in older Latinos are poor, in part due to the underutilization of mental health services by this group and high rates of dropout in studies related to psychotherapeutic treatment.[19] A primary concept important to Latinos includes the idea of "familismo," in which their identities are formed based on their understanding of themselves and their connections with family and others. As such, the Western, individualistic style of psychotherapy may conflict with what might be more appropriate for the sociocentric-minded culture seen in Latinos.[20] For example, adaptation and incorporation of more culture-specific beliefs and values in cognitive behavioral therapy (CBT) can help modify treatment targeting more culture-specific strengths and coping skills to create the desired behavioral changes.[21,22] For Latinos, some have argued that a behavioral approach may better target some key issues for older Latinos, including the acculturation process, socio-economic difficulties, prejudicial treatment from others, and changing roles within the family setting, compared to a more cognitive approach.[19] Because of the limited evidence for therapy modality, what seems more important than approach is focus on treatment engagement and retention using culturally sensitive and appropriate therapeutic strategies.

Evidence for psychotherapy with older African Americans is sorely lacking; however, work done with African American adults can help inform work with older adults. Culturally sensitive strategies to incorporate into psychotherapy include an understanding of African American history and racial identity; an appreciation of the role of institutionalized racism in limiting individual agency of African Americans; and the complex relationship between the institutions of power, such as the legal and judicial systems, and individual African Americans.[23] Psychotherapists should pay special attention to the therapeutic alliance, as previous experiences of bias and discrimination can affect African Americans' ability to develop strong therapeutic alliances.[24] Research has also identified internalized stigma as a particularly challenging barrier for older African Americans.[25] Unfortunately, there is limited information on the efficacy of specific therapy techniques. Psychoeducation about psychotherapy has led to higher rates of attendance and a more positive outlook on therapy experiences in older African Americans[26] and should be incorporated into clinical practice to encourage engagement in psychotherapy. Problem-solving therapy has been shown to reduce the incidence of depression in African Americans with subsyndromal symptoms,[27] as has other multimodal, practical psychotherapy.[28]

Many Asian American immigrant groups come from backgrounds where there is little education or exposure to mental health and treatment. Because there are cultural differences in presentation of illness, such as the tendency to report more somatic symptoms and the tendency not to report psychological symptoms, as well as stigma associated with mental health treatment, there has been lower treatment usage and help-seeking among Asian American patients.[16] Sharing weakness and emotional distress has also been viewed unfavorably, especially for older Asian American patients. Brief, focused, problem-based therapy may be more effective in older Asian Americans, who might be resistant to the self-disclosure involved in insight-oriented psychotherapy.[7] Challenges related to the trauma of immigration, a bicultural sense of self, and acculturation may emerge as themes in treatment.[14]

In traditional psychoanalytic psychotherapy, in particular, Asian patients generally observe the social etiquette of formal hierarchies in which they are expected to show deference, respect, and obedience to their superiors, keeping disagreements and negative feelings to themselves. This inherent sense of respect and obedience makes it especially challenging to address challenges related to anger and hate in psychotherapy, since patients may try to sense what the therapist expects of them rather than freely discussing negative transference.[14] Psychotherapists can and should help patients broaden their perspective on how to improve the helping relationship and recognize the therapist's ability to engage in more effective psychotherapy.[16]

Other cultural aspects to consider are intragroup variances in education, socioeconomic status, and careers. Asians in general are stereotyped into the "model minority" and portrayed as working hard, being highly educated, and having higher incomes than the general population. However, these overgeneralizations neglect individual variance. Socioeconomic problems and cultural expectations of accomplishment should be explored, as these can be prominent underlying stressors that may not be evident or disclosed during therapy.[29,30]

In sum, helpful considerations to address race and ethnicity in psychotherapy include the following: (1) suspending preconceptions about the patients' race/ethnicity and that of their family members; (2) recognizing that patients may be different from other members of their racial/ethnic group; (3) considering how racial/ethnic differences between the therapist and the patient may affect psychotherapy; (4) acknowledging that power, privilege, and racism may affect interactions with patients; and (5) discussing race and ethnicity in the treatment when in doubt about its importance.[31] The ability to conduct psychotherapy effectively with racially and ethnically diverse older adults is becoming increasingly important given the changing demographics of the United States. Cultural issues constitute key elements in psychotherapy and can even touch deep unconscious feelings for both patient and therapist. Acknowledging these differences can serve as catalysts to address multicultural therapeutic issues that strengthen the therapeutic alliance and promote better treatment outcomes.

Women

Older adults are the nation's fastest growing cohort, with the majority being older women. In 2050, 55% of adults aged 65 and older and 62% of adults aged 85 and over will be women.[32] When psychoanalytic and psychodynamic theories dominated the field of psychotherapy, women would often somaticize their emotional pain through physical ailments and were described as passive, dependent, and morally inferior to men.[33] Although there have been a number of modifications and innovations to therapy approaches, psychological problems that continue to have a higher prevalence in women include problems of marital and family relations, reproductive problems, physical and sexual abuse, depression, and problems associated with eating. For older women, challenges emerge related to menopause, retirement, caregiving, and widowhood. Additionally, cultural attitudes about the meaning of menopause, as well as socioeconomic realities, work opportunities, sexual beliefs, and health status can all contribute to how a woman experiences older age.[34]

Although some literature examines gender differences and psychotherapy outcomes, less is understood about these differences for older women. In the past decades, systematic research exploring gender-related responses to psychotherapy have yielded mixed and inconsistent results. Men may benefit more from individual interpretive therapy than from supportive therapy, and women vice versa.[35] Women seem to have superior responses to both interpretive and group therapy compared to men. Taken together, these findings suggest that women prefer a more collaborative, personal approach in psychotherapy.[36] More recent reviews, however, have found no impact of gender on psychotherapy responses.[37,38]

Women are particularly vulnerable to poverty, discrimination, violence, and marginalization in old age. Additional gender-related vulnerabilities among older women include limited socialization, prevalence of domestic violence, lower socioeconomic status, sexism, oppression, and adverse portrayal in society and the media.[39] Traditional gender roles in the United States and Western European countries assumed that a woman's primary involvement in society was reproductive labor, unpaid housework, and caregiving. Uncompensated caregiving activities often restricted women's social mobility, educational attainment, and skills development, thereby limiting their employment and earning opportunities.[40] Even when women entered the work force, they earned less and saved less for their elderly years than men.[39] Most older women are dependent on Social Security as their primary income, with only half receiving any type of pension payments.[41] Although the majority of women are not considered impoverished when their husbands die, many fall into poverty with age. Roughly 75% of older adults who fall within the poverty level are women.[41]

Caregiving of spouses is often much more stressful for elderly women than men. Many women remain overburdened and less likely to ask for help, as requesting assistance may feel like an abdication of their female responsibilities. Similarly, many women are unable to enjoy their later years because they struggle to meet their basic needs both physically and financially.[39,42] Increased life expectancy for women also means they are faced with a longer period of potential disability. A National Long-Term Care Study with data from 1984, 1989, and 1994 indicated that 30% of the residual life expectancy at age 65 for women was spent in a state of chronic disability. As older women confront the greater dependence that comes with the breakdown of body systems, therapists may help clarify the advantages of "inter-dependence" in order for women to maintain an intact sense of self. Key therapeutic approaches may also be working to support and empower women in these new role transitions to facilitate dignity, self-fulfillment, and equality.[34] According to prior research, several nonspecific factors, such as the quality of the therapeutic alliance, severity of the patient's psychological problems, and the therapist's competence and experience, may be more important than the impact of gender on specific therapy modalities or outcomes.[35,38] Understanding gender issues and the cumulative effects of these gender disparities across a woman's life is key to developing a sustainable working alliance.

Lesbian, Gay, Bisexual, Transgender, and Queer Older Adults

There are at least 1.5 million lesbian, gay, and bisexual adults aged 65 and over currently living in the United States.[43] How many individuals identify as transgender is harder to estimate, but the number is likely to grow as acceptance of transgender and the population of gender-nonconforming individuals grows. Despite being part of a growing population of older adults, lesbian, gay, bisexual, transgender, and queer (LGBTQ) individuals remain less frequently studied in empirical research, and the specific evidence base for psychotherapy with LGBTQ older adults remains poor.

For many older adults, the experience of growing up as a LGBTQ individual in a society with few protections created significant internalized homophobia. A strong desire for acceptance from authority figures and peers conflicted with their own sexual desires, resulting in shame and secrecy.[44,45] Treatments such as affirmative psychotherapy developed specifically for work around identity acceptance with LGBTQ populations are helpful in reducing the painful emotions associated with LGBTQ identity for many older adults.[46] As LGBTQ adults move into skilled nursing and assisted living facilities with peers they had worked to avoid, they again may be confronted with homophobia and transphobia.

Psychotherapy with all adults often focuses on restarting development. With older LGBTQ adults, many adult milestones, particularly around marriage, career, and family, can be significantly delayed because of stigma, shame, discrimination, or some combination of the three.[44,45,47] Good psychotherapy includes consideration of age-appropriate life goals, and working with older LGBTQ adults may mean adjusting what is considered age-appropriate, in particular maintaining a nonpathologic viewpoint on delays in psychosexual development. LGBTQ older adults may have fewer romantic and sexual relationships than their non-LGBTQ peers.[43]

Cultural events and shifts also affect LGBTQ seniors differently than non-LGBTQ seniors. For many gay men, movement to cities in the late 1960s and 1970s coincided with a sexual awakening, often involving nonmonogamous relationships and casual sex. These mores shifted following the AIDS crisis of the 1980s, in which many gay and bisexual men died from AIDS. For those who survived, the guilt of living while so many died cannot be understated and may color psychotherapeutic work with older LGBTQ individuals.[47] The legalization of marriage between two individuals of the same sex has proved to be another major milestone, and will undoubtedly create cohort effects in future LGBTQ older adults, some of whom may be opposed to the heteronormativity of marriage.[44,45,47]

Finally, the intersectionality inherent in working with any diverse population will be magnified when working with LGBTQ older adults. By being both older and LGBTQ, they already maintain status as belonging to two groups facing discrimination. For those adults who identify as a third or even fourth marginalized group, understanding the interrelated and perhaps conflicting feelings about membership in multiple identity groups can make for challenging, yet also rewarding, psychotherapeutic work.

Veterans

Older veterans present with a unique set of challenges. High incidences of post-traumatic stress disorder (PTSD), military sexual trauma, traumatic brain injury (TBI), and comorbid substance use present distinctive clinical presentations that can be complex and difficult to treat. While Veterans Health Administration (VHA) centers around the country offer extensive services for veterans, individual practitioners may find themselves providing psychotherapy for older veterans in the community.

Current guidelines have been published by the VA and Department of Defense for the treatment of commonly seen disorders in the veteran population. For example, first-line treatment for mild to moderate major depressive disorder (MDD) includes pharmacological interventions and/or evidence-based psychotherapy modalities, including CBT, acceptance and commitment therapy (ACT), behavioral activation (BA), interpersonal psychotherapy (IPT), problem-solving therapy (PST), and mindfulness-based cognitive therapy.[48] For patients with primary or comorbid PTSD, there is strong evidence for individual trauma-focused therapies that have as a principal piece cognitive restructuring and trauma exposure.[49] These include but are not limited to cognitive processing therapy, prolonged exposure, narrative exposure therapy, and eye movement desensitization and reprocessing. Overall, psychotherapy was preferred over pharmacological treatments as first-line treatment for PTSD symptoms.[49] Among these types of therapy, prolonged exposure therapy has been specifically tested in the older veterans' population with promising results.[50] Older veterans with comorbid substance use benefit from relapse prevention interventions with CBT; this combined approach has been shown to improve abstinence outcomes in senior veterans.[51] Motivational enhancement therapy and 12-step facilitation also have a strong evidence base for treatment in comorbid substance abuse.[52]

As with other older adults, veterans' access to therapy can be limited due to a variety of circumstances including financial and medical constraints, and impaired mobility. Preliminary studies on telemedicine-based psychotherapy for older veterans with depression have shown outcomes similar to those with patients receiving same-room treatment.[53] Telemedicine-based psychotherapy may become an acceptable alternative for veterans who are unable to utilize same-room treatment due to lack of accessibility.[53]

Conclusion

More research is needed to identify optimal psychotherapeutic approaches to successfully engage and treat diverse older adults. Although specific guidance on evidence-based psychotherapies is limited, some specific challenges outlined in this chapter offer a starting point for practitioners to consider when providing psychotherapy to older adults. The type of psychotherapy treatment may be less important than the psychotherapist's comfort in addressing the difficult issues facing diverse older adults. As the United States population continues to age, understanding the specific challenges faced by diverse older adults will become essential to all psychotherapists.

References

1. Blazer DG, Steffens DC. Treatment of seniors. In: Hales RE, Yudofsky SC, Roberts LW, editors. *Textbook of psychiatry*. 6th ed. Arlington, VA: American Psychiatric Publishing; 2014. p. 1233–1262.

2. Lu FG, Lewis-Fernandez R, Primm AB, Lim RF, Aggarwal NK. Treatment of culturally diverse populations. In: Hales RE, Yudofsky SC, Roberts LW, editors. *Textbook of psychiatry*. 6th ed. Arlington, VA: American Psychiatric Publishing; 2014. p. 1263–1292.

3. Passel J, Livingston G, Cohn D. Explaining why minority births now outnumber white births. *Pew Social and Demographic Trends. Pew Research Center*; 2012. Retrieved from: www.pewsocialtrends.org/2012/05/17/ explaining-why-minority-births-now-outnumber-white-births (November 2018).

4. American Psychiatric Association DSM-5 Cultural Formulation Interview (CFI); 2013. Retrieved from: www.psychiatry.org/ File%20Library/Psychiatrists/Practice/ DSM/APA_DSM5_Cultural-Formulation-Interview.pdf (December 2018).

5. Falicov CJ. Changing constructions of machismo for Latino men in therapy: "the devil never sleeps." *Family Process*. 2010;**49**(3):309–329.

6. Paniagua FA, Yamada AM, editors. *Handbook of multicultural mental health: assessment and treatment of diverse populations*. 2nd ed. San Diego, CA: Elsevier; 2013.

7. Leong FT, Lee SH. A cultural accommodation model for cross-cultural psychotherapy: illustrated with the case of Asian Americans. *Psychotherapy: Theory, Research, Practice, Training*. 2006;**43**(4):410–423.

8. Ryder NB. The cohort as a concept in the study of social change. *Am Sociol Rev*. 1965;**30**(6):843–861.

9. Pan D, Huey SJ Jr, Hernandez D. Culturally adapted versus standard exposure treatment for phobic Asian Americans: treatment efficacy, moderators, and predictors. *Cultur Divers Ethnic Minor Psychol*. 2011;**17**(1):11–22.

10. Karlsson R. Ethnic matching between therapist and patient in psychotherapy: an overview of findings, together with methodological and conceptual issues. *Cultur Divers Ethnic Minor Psychol*. 2005;**11**:113–129.

11. Cabral RR, Smith TB. Racial/ethnic matching of clients and therapists in mental health services: a meta-analytic review of preferences, perceptions, and outcomes. *J Couns Psychol*. 2011;**58**(4):537–554.

12. Presnell A, Harris G, Scogin F. Therapist and client race/ethnicity match: an examination of treatment outcomes and process with rural older adults in the Deep South. *Psychother Res*. 2012;**22**(4):458–463.

13. Meghani SH, Brooks JM, Gipson-Jones T, et al. Patient–provider race-concordance: does it matter in improving minority patients' health outcomes? *Ethn Health*. 2009;**14**(1):107–130.

14. Roland A. Across civilizations: psychoanalytic therapy with Asians and Asian Americans. *Psychotherapy: Theory, Research, Practice, Training*. 2006;**43**(4):454–463.

15. Benish SG, Quintana S, Wampold BE. Culturally adapted psychotherapy and the legitimacy of myth: a direct-comparison meta-analysis. *J Couns Psychol*. 2011;**58**(3):279–289.

16. Hwang WC. The psychotherapy adaptation and modification framework. *Application*

to Asian Americans. *American Psychologist.* 2006;**61**(7):702–715.

17. Jimenez DE, Bartels SJ, Cardenas V, Dhaliwal SS, Alegria M. Cultural beliefs and mental health treatment preferences of ethnically diverse older adult consumers in primary care. *Am J Geriatr Psychiatry.* 2012;**20**(6):533–542.

18. Comas-Diaz L, Jacobsen FM. Ethnocultural transference and countertransference in the therapeutic dyad. *Am J Orthopsychial.* 1991; **61**(3):392–402.

19. Santiago-Rivera A, Kanter J, Benson G, et al. Behavioral activation as an alternative treatment approach for Latinos with depression. *Psychotherapy: Theory, Research, Practice, Training.* 2008;**45** (2):173–185.

20. Comas-Diaz L. The future of psychotherapy with ethnic minorities. *Psychotherapy Theory Research & Practice.* 1992;**29**(1):88–94.

21. Hays PA. Multicultural applications of cognitive-behavior therapy. *Professional Psychology: Research and Practice.* 1995;**26** (3):309–315.

22. Sue S. Psychotherapeutic services for ethnic minorities: two decades of research findings. *American Psychologist.* 1988;**43** (4):301–308.

23. Thorn GR, Sarata BP. Psychotherapy with African American men: what we know and what we need to know. *J Multicult Couns Devel.* 1998;**26**(4):240–253.

24. Thompson VLS, Bazile A, Akbar M. African Americans' perceptions of psychotherapy and psychotherapists. *Prof Psychol Res Pr.* 2004;**35**(1):19–26.

25. Conner KO, Copeland VC, Grote NK, et al. Barriers to treatment and culturally endorsed coping strategies among depressed African-American older adults. *Aging Ment Health.* 2010;**14**(8):971–983.

26. Alvidrez J, Areán PA, Stewart AL. Psychoeducation to increase psychotherapy entry for older African Americans. *Am J Geriatr Psychiatry.* 2005;**13**(7):554–561.

27. Reynolds CF 3rd, Thomas SB, Morse JQ, et al. Early interventions to preempt major

depression among older black and white adults. *Psychiatric Services.* 2014;**65** (6):765–773.

28. Gitlin LN, Szanton SL, Huang J, Roth DL. Factors mediating the effects of a depression intervention on functional disability in older African Americans. *J Am Geriatr Soc.* 2014;**62**(12):2280–2287.

29. Kim BJ, Sangalang CC, Kihl T. Effects of acculturation and social network support on depression among elderly Korean immigrants. *Aging Ment Health.* 2012;**16** (6):787–794.

30. Paniagua FA, editor. *Handbook of multicultural mental health: assessment and treatment of diverse populations.* San Diego, CA: Elsevier; 2000.

31. Cardemil EV, Battle CL. Guess who's coming to therapy? Getting comfortable with conversations about race and ethnicity in psychotherapy. *Prof Psychol Res Pr.* 2003;**34**(3):278–286.

32. Ortman JM, Velkoff VA, Hogan H. *An aging nation: the older population in the United States.* US Census Bureau Current Population Reports; 2014.

33. Hare-Mustin RT. An appraisal of the relationship between women and psychotherapy. 80 years after the case of Dora. *Am Psychol.* 1983;**38**(5):593–601.

34. Trotman FK, Brody C, with contributors. *Psychotherapy and counseling with older women, cross-cultural, family, and end-of-life issues.* New York: Springer; 2002.

35. Ogrodniczuk JS, Piper WE, Joyce AS, McCallum M. Effect of gender on outcome in two forms of short term individual psychotherapy. *J Psychother Pract Res.* 2001;**10**:69–78.

36. Ogrodniczuk JS. Men, women, and their outcome in psychotherapy. *Psychother Res.* 2006;**16**:453–462.

37. Parker G, Blanch B, Crawford J. Does gender influence response to differing psychotherapies by those with unipolar depression? *J Affect Disord.* 2011;**130**:17–20.

38. Staczan P, Schmuecker R, Koehler M, et al. Effects of sex and gender in ten types of

psychotherapy. *Psychother Res.* 2017;**27** (1):74–88.

39. Steuer JL. Psychotherapy with older women: ageism and sexism in traditional practice. *Psychotherapy: Theory, Research, and Practice.* 1982;**19**(4):429–436.

40. Mlambo-Ngcuka P. Challenges facing older women: the feminization of aging. Women's UN Report Network; 2017. Retrieved from: wunrn.com/2017/02/challenges-facing-older-women-the-feminization-of-aging/ (October 2018).

41. World Population Data Population Reference Bureau; 2018. Retrieved from: www.worldpopdata.org/ (October 2018).

42. Brown JE, Rhee N, Saad-Lessler J, Oakley D. Shortchanged in retirement: continuing challenges to women's financial retirement. National Institute on Retirement Security; 2016. Retrieved from: www.nirsonline.org/wp-content/uploads/2017/06/final_shortchanged_retirement_report_2016.pdf (October 2018).

43. Grant JM, Kosovich G, Frazer MS, Bjerk S, SAGE. Outing age 2010: public policy issues affecting gay, lesbian, bisexual and transgender elders. 2010. Retrieved from: www.thetaskforce.org/downloads/reports/reports/outingage_final.pdf (November 2018).

44. Hash KM, Rogers A. Clinical practice with older LGBT clients: overcoming lifelong stigma through strength and resilience. *Clin Soc Work J.* 2013;**41**:249–257.

45. Steven D, Cernin PA. Psychotherapy with lesbian, gay, bisexual, and transgender older adults. *J Gay Lesbian Soc Serv.* 2008;**20**:31–49.

46. Hinrichs KLM, Donaldson W. Recommendations for use of affirmative psychotherapy with LGBT older adults. *J Clin Psychol.* 2017;**73**:945–953.

47. Fredriksen-Goldsen KI, Hoy-Ellis CP, Goldsen J, Emlet CA, Hooyman NR. Creating a vision for the future: key competencies and strategies for culturally competent practice with lesbian, gay, bisexual, and transgender (LGBT) older adults in the health and human services. *J Gerontol Soc Work.* 2014;**57** (24):80–107.

48. Management of MDD Working Group. *VA/DoD clinical practice guideline for management of major depressive disorder (MDD).* Washington, DC: Department of Defense, Department of Veterans Affairs; 2016. Retrieved from: www.healthquality.va.gov/guidelines/MH/mdd/VADoDMDDCPGFINAL82916.pdf (October 2018).

49. The Management of Post-Traumatic Stress Working Group. *VA/DoD clinical practice guideline for management of post-traumatic stress.* Washington, DC: Department of Defense, Department of Veterans Affairs; 2017. Retrieved from: www.healthquality.va.gov/guidelines/MH/ptsd/VADoDPTSDCPGFinal012418.pdf (October 2018).

50. Thorp SR, Stein MB, Jeste DV, Patterson TL, Wetherell JL. Prolonged exposure therapy for older veterans with posttraumatic stress disorder: a pilot study. *Am J Geriatr Psychiatry.* 2012;**20** (3):276–280.

51. Schonfeld L, Dupree LW, Dickson-Fuhrmann E, et al. Cognitive-behavioral treatment of older veterans with substance abuse problems. *J Geriatr Psychiatry Neurol.* 2000;**13**(3):124–129.

52. Management of Substance Use Disorders Working Group. *VA/DoD clinical practice guideline for management of substance use disorders (SUD).* Washington, DC: Department of Defense, Department of Veterans Affairs; 2015. Retrieved from: www.healthquality.va.gov/guidelines/MH/sud/VADODSUDCPGRevised22216.pdf (October 2018).

53. Egede LE, Acierno R, Knapp RG, et al. Psychotherapy for depression in older veterans via telemedicine: a randomised, open-label, non-inferiority trial. *The Lancet Psychiatry.* 2015;**2**(8):693–701.

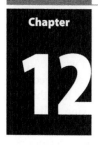

Chapter

12

Individual versus Group Psychotherapy

Paroma Mitra

Introduction

By the year 2030, projections suggest that the number of older adults will be greater than the number of people younger than 18. This number will exceed 98 million by 2050.[1] Community studies from Europe and North America suggest that depressive symptoms may be seen among 30–45% of older adults,[2–4] and symptoms of anxiety among 15–20%.[4] A significant portion of older adults (about 15%) has ongoing cognitive symptomatology.[5]

The previous chapters in this book have described treatment approaches by individual therapy, and among older adults who receive any form of therapy the majority does receive individual therapy. Group therapy has not been extensively studied in older adults;[6] however, several small randomized controlled trials (RCTs) have been done in this population. A recent systemic review assessed the evidence for group therapy among nine international studies and concluded that both reminiscence therapy (RT) and cognitive behavioral therapy (CBT) were effective for late-life depression.[7] This chapter will highlight these methods of group therapy used for older adults as well as the use of group therapy for cognitively impaired patients, and will discuss the evidence available for use of each approach.

Introduction to the Concept of Group Therapy

Group therapy is an evidence-based treatment that involves a small number of people and one or more therapists who are trained in both group and individual therapy.[8,9] Group therapy was developed in the early 1900s around the concept of pragmatism, or the idea that identity is shaped by environment. In this way, people are affected by the systems they inhabit.[9] This approach traditionally uses interactions among group members and the therapist(s) to mitigate certain target symptoms.[9] Some studies have shown in the general population that group therapy is cost-effective and as effective as individual therapy.[10,11] Such findings, however, have not yet been replicated specifically in older adults.

Group Cognitive Behavioral Therapy for Anxiety and Depression

Group CBT is helpful for older adults presenting with symptoms of depression and anxiety.[8,12] In an older adult population, chronic physical impairments often contribute to these psychological symptoms.[13] Group CBT provides a format in which older adults may speak with others undergoing similar physical and psychological stressors, and this, in particular, may be beneficial for those who are otherwise socially isolated.[13,14] Group CBT is also suited for older adults who have experienced loss of family and social support, as groups provide the additional benefit of a social support system.[15]

A few RCTs have overall shown advantages of group CBT in international settings in the community. For example, a group in China demonstrated a positive effect for group CBT in older Chinese adults with generalized anxiety disorder (GAD).[16] The largest study published was in Australia and looked at group CBT for anxiety and depression with 133 participants in the community. A positive effect was seen in the initial month compared to a non-structured group; however, this difference became insignificant in six months.[13,17] Improvements in executive functioning, processing speed, and problem-solving skills have been demonstrated in some studies as well.[18,19] It is difficult to synthesize the overall benefit of group CBT across these cultures and extrapolate to others due to varying recruitment strategies, methodologies, and cultural influences.[17,20]

Framework of Group Cognitive Behavioral Therapy

Larry Thompson's guide to CBT lays out the basic skeletal framework for which group CBT may be conducted in older adults.[21]

Assessment: The first step is an individual assessment interview. Assessing eligibility of persons to participate in the group is vital. This includes addressing any sensory impairments (e.g., hearing and vision loss), mobility limitations, and access to transportation. The group leader must have access to the medical and psychiatric history of each patient. Ideally, assessment scales are completed prior to starting group therapy. Regular depression scales such as Beck's Depression Inventory (BDI) or the Geriatric Depression Scale (GDS) may be used.[21,22] Another scale that may be useful before starting group work may be the Older Person's Pleasant Events Schedule. This is a list of 66 items that people tend to find pleasant. For every question, the frequency is measured on a Likert Scale ranging from 0–2. The intensity is also measured from 0–2.[23]

Preparing the Group: The framework of CBT is laid out in the first session and includes setting the frame, introducing problem-solving, and explaining homework. The number of sessions is ideally 10–12, each for 90 minutes. Before commencing therapy, it may be helpful to explain basic concepts of therapy in the group. Usually participants are asked to identify 2–3 issues that each may want to address.[12,14]

Structure of sessions: Each session typically begins with reviewing homework from the previous session. Group members problem-solve with each other and are encouraged to bring up challenges from the assigned homework. Group members reach consensus on the day's agenda. Mindfulness exercises and relaxation techniques may be taught through the sessions.[14] The end of the session focuses on homework or behavioral techniques that need to be worked on before the next meeting. As sessions progress, homework may differ as well for each group member. Group members are encouraged to use creative techniques in this process.[12]

Tools to be used: Several tools may be helpful for monitoring patients between sessions. A mood monitoring tool, such a daily mood rating form, may be used by group members to assess progress. Examples of rating scales may include a 9-point Likert scale that patients use to identify their daily numeric rating of mood (e.g., a range from 0–9 ranging from very depressed to very happy). The standard Patient Health Questionnaire (PHQ-9) may be used as a weekly questionnaire.[24] Many mobile applications can chart mood changes and can be taught to older adults as well. For example, Posit Science is one of the many applications that charts mood daily.[25] All participants would be expected to maintain a daily record of unhelpful thoughts as per standard CBT protocol.[26] An activities scale, including pleasurable activities and tasks needing to be mastered, may be maintained through the week as well. The principles and framework of Group CBT have been derived largely from Beck's principles of cognitive behavioral therapy.[26]

Group Reminiscence Therapy

Reminiscence therapy means "using the recall of past events, feelings, and thoughts to facilitate pleasure, quality of life, or adaptation to present circumstances of self-esteem through confirmation of their uniqueness."[27] Reminiscence group therapy involves the vocal or silent recall of past events of life.[28] This form of therapy encourages discussion of past events in a person's life with the help of prompts.[29] The benefits of RT with other adults include its help with spontaneous conversation, emotional stimulation, and promotion of self-esteem.[29] It can also be used with people experiencing moderate to severe neurocognitive disorder. The three types of RT include simple reminiscence, life review, and life-review therapy. Simple reminiscence emphasizes social stimulation and enhances connections among group members. Life review uses memories and past problem-solving skills to integrate into the present self. Life-review therapy addresses present negativistic coping skills to specifically target aspects of ongoing mental distress.[30]

Several studies of RT have shown positive outcomes for older adults for mood, well-being, anxiety, cohesiveness, and quality of life.[31–33] A number of international studies conducted in the community have shown overall reduction in depressive symptoms in late-life depression by using group RT, particularly life-review therapy.[33,34] Some similar controlled trials, however, have been inconclusive.[35,36]

A few studies have shown the benefits of reminiscence for patients with cognitive impairment (CI). One prospective study in Asia showed an overall positive effect on cognitive functions among patients with Alzheimer's disease (AD).[33] A study in Turkey examined the effect of RT on patients with AD residing in a nursing home. Overall, there were positive effects on cognitive function, depressive symptoms, and quality of life.[32] A meta-analysis that assembled data on twelve RCTs demonstrated a small-size benefit on cognitive functions and depressive symptoms for a short period of time. Participants were followed for 6–10 months. Long-term effects were not confirmed. The meta-analysis advocated for RT to be offered as part of routine care for persons with dementia.[37]

A few quasi-RCTs in long-term care facilities looked at reduction in feelings of loneliness using reminiscence therapy.[38–40] One review summarized 8 trials with a total of 100 participants in long-term care facilities using group RT and concluded that there has not been adequate evidence to determine whether group RT was effective in reducing loneliness in older adults in long-term care facilities.[36] The authors did not make conclusions about reduction in symptoms of depression or anxiety, given that the approaches to treatment differed widely among sites.[36]

Framework of Approach

Few texts exist on the use of RT, and most of them concern working with older adults and often describe the use of RT in a group format.[27,41] Participants include not only patients but also their caregivers and other staff. Reminiscence therapy may be conducted in inpatient, outpatient, or residential settings. Delivery of therapy largely varies depending on the participants and issues faced by the group.[42]

Reminiscence therapy groups are structured with approximately 8–12 sessions. The first session serves as an introduction and the last session as a goodbye/evaluation session. Prior to the start of the group, facilitators identify the main goals (such as social stimulation or cognitive rehabilitation). Facilitators may want to anticipate that more participants will join than originally planned. Themes explored in this type of therapy may include significant historical events that occurred during the participants' lifetimes, relationships, and meaningful locations. Facilitators may also wish to collaborate with caregivers and other team members to identify subjects that should be avoided.[27,36]

Group Therapy for Cognitive Impairment

Forms of sensory therapy (like art and music) have been shown to have multiple benefits for patients with cognitive impairment.[43,44] Cohen-Mansfield's group has explored the framework of how patients with dementia interact with the environment.[45,46] Studies have shown that even brief social interaction is stimulating for people with dementia.[47] Although many of these therapeutic approaches may be conducted in a residential or group setting, limited treatment guidelines exist for group therapy among older adults with cognitive impairment. A small number of RCTs have been conducted outside the United States. A study in China of patients with mild cognitive impairment (MCI) in long-term facilities found that use of reminiscence group therapy improved cognitive functions.[48] Another group in the Netherlands studied group CBT for patients with MCI and their partners for 6–8 months. There were increased depressive symptoms and hopelessness in the group with MCI, but patients demonstrated better insight.[49]

A recent paper by the Cohen-Mansfield group introduced a theoretical model that involved therapeutic group activities for engaging patients with dementia.[50] Some activities suggested included reading, baking, creative storytelling, brain games/fitness, active games, exercise, poetry, creation of a holiday newsletter, and discussions on health.[51] They presented a framework to accommodate challenges in this population, such as attendance and alertness. In nursing homes and other long-term care facilities that often house people with CI, group therapy has benefits such as increased socialization, improved communication, and formation of new connections within facilities.[52]

Support Groups for Caregivers

Older adults frequently serve in the role of caregiver, with recipients of care including their own aging parents, partners, children, or grandchildren. Caregiving responsibilities can be physically and emotionally demanding, and many caregivers suffer from burnout.[53] They may present with poor functioning, mood lability, anxiety, or guilt.[54] Support groups may be helpful for caregivers to target these symptoms. These groups are often psychoeducational in nature and emphasize the development of coping skills.[57] Interventions such as relaxation training and mindfulness may be helpful components of support groups.[55-57] Research is limited regarding the use of support groups among older adult caregivers, and thus these strategies are extrapolated from research in groups for a broader adult age range.

Conclusions

Studies exploring the use of group therapy in older adults are limited; however, a few randomized trials have shown fair outcomes, especially for older adults experiencing depression, anxiety, and cognitive impairment. The most common approaches to group therapy in older adults include group CBT and reminiscence therapy. Some research examining the benefit of support groups for caregivers of all ages may apply to the older-adult population. As of the time of this publication, no studies had examined use of group therapy for treatment of late-life psychosis or substance use. Lack of standardized approaches to therapy among the few RCTs conducted has led to limited understanding of group therapy among older adults. More research evaluating the role of group therapy for older adults is imperative in light of the rapid growth of the aging population.

References

1. U.S. Census Bureau. National population projections: summary tables. US Census Website; 2014. Retrieved from: www.census.gov/population/projections/data/national/2014/summarytables.html

2. Copeland JR, Beekman AT, Braam AW, et al. Depression among older people in Europe: the EURODEP studies. *World Psychiatry*. 2004;**3**:45–49.

3. Alexopoulos GS. Depression in the elderly. *Lancet*. 2005;**365**(9475):1961–1970.

4. Reynold K, Pietrzak RH, El-Gabalawy R, et al. Prevalence of psychiatric disorders in U.S. older adults: findings from a nationally representative survey. *World Psychiatry*. 2015;**14**(1):74–81.

5. Hurd MD, Martorell P, Delavande A, et al. Monetary costs of dementia in the United States. *N Engl J Med*. 2013;**368**:1326–1334.

6. Huang AX, Delucchi K, Dunn LB, et al. A systematic review and meta-analysis of psychotherapy for late-life depression. *Am J Geriatric Psychiatry*. 2015;**23**(3):261–273.

7. Tavares LR, Barbosa MR. Efficacy of group psychotherapy for geriatric depression: a systemic review. *Arch Gerontol Geriatric*. 2018;**78**:71–80.

8. Arean PA, Smoski MJ. Individual and group therapy. In: Steffens DC, Blazer DG, Thakur ME, editors. *The American psychiatric publishing textbook of geriatric psychiatry*. Fifth ed. Washington, DC: American Psychiatric Publishing; 2015.

9. Brabender V, Fallon, AE, Smolar, AI. *Essentials of group therapy*. Hoboken, NY: John Wiley & Sons; 1998. Chapter 1: Introduction to group therapy.

10. Brown JS, Sellwood K, Beecham JK, et al. Outcome, costs and patient engagement for group and individual CBT for depression: a naturalistic clinical study. *Behav Cogn Psychotherapy*. 2011;**39**(3):355–358.

11. Bland P. Group CBT is a cost-effective option for persistent back pain. *Practitioner*. 2010;**254**(1728):7.

12. Thompson L, Powers D, Coon D, et al. Psychotherapy with older people. In: Older adults. Cognitive behavioral group therapy: for specific problems and populations; 2000.

13. McLaughlin DP, McFarland K. A randomized trial of a group based cognitive behavior therapy program for older adults with epilepsy: the impact on seizure frequency, depression and psychosocial well-being. *J Behav Med*. 2011;**34**(3):201–207.

14. Dick LP, Gallagher-Thompson D, Coon DW, et al. *Cognitive-behavioral therapy for late-life depression: a client manual*. Palo Alto, CA: Veterans Affairs Palo Alto Health Care System; 1996.

15. Areán PA. Cognitive behavioral therapy with older adults. *The Behavior Therapist*. 1993;**16**(9):236–239.

16. Chen H, Yang Z. Group cognitive behavioral therapy targeting intolerance of uncertainty: a randomized trial for older Chinese adults with generalized anxiety disorder. *Aging Ment Health*. 2017;**21**(12):1294–1302.

17. Wuthrich VM, Rapee R, Kangas M, et al. Randomized controlled trial of group cognitive behavioral therapy compared to a discussion group for co-morbid anxiety and depression in older adults. *Psychol Med*. 2016;**46**:785–795.

18. Jonsson U, Bertilsson G, Allerd P, et al. Psychological treatment of depression in people aged 65 years and over: a systematic review of efficacy, safety, and cost-effectiveness. *PLoS ONE*. 2016;**11**(8).

19. Simon SS, Cordas TA, Bottino CM. Cognitive behavioral therapies in older adults with depression and cognitive deficits: a systematic review. *Int J Geriatr Psychiatry*. 2015;30:223–233.

20. García-Peña C, Vázquez-Estupiñan F, Avalos-Pérez F,et al. Clinical effectiveness of group cognitive behavioral therapy for depressed older people in primary care: a randomized controlled trial. *Salud Mental*. 2015;38(1):33–39.

21. Beck AT, Ward CH, Mendelson M., et al. An inventory for measuring depression. *Arch Gen Psychiatry*. 1961;4:561–571.

22 Brink TL, Yesavage JA, Lum O, et al. Screening tests for geriatric depression. *Clin Gerontol*. 1982;1:7–43.

23. Rider KL, Thompson L, Gallagher-Thompson D. California older persons pleasant events scale: a tool to help older adults increase positive experiences. *COPPES – Clin Gerontol*. 2016;39(1):64–83.

24. Kronke K, Williams J, Spitzer RL. The PHQ-9 validity of a brief depression severity measure. *J Gen Intern Med*. 2001;16(9):606–613.

25. Nahum M, Van Vleet TM, Sohal VS. Immediate mood scaler: tracking symptoms of depression and anxiety using a novel mobile mood scale. *JMIR Mhealth & Uhealth*. 2017;5(4):e44.

26. Beck JS. *Cognitive behavior therapy: Basics and beyond*. 2nd ed. New York: Guilford Press; 2011.

27. Bender M, Bauckham P, Norris A. *The therapeutic purposes of reminiscence*. London: Sage; 1998.

28. Cotelli M, Manenti R, Zanetti O. Reminiscence therapy in dementia: a review. *Maturitas*. 2012;72(3):203–205.

29. Pinquart M, Forstmeier S. Effects of reminiscence interventions on psychosocial outcomes: a meta-analysis. *Aging Ment Health*. 2012;16(5):541–558.

30. Westerhof GJ, Bohlmeijer E, Webster JD. Reminiscence and mental health: a review of recent progress in theory, research and interventions. *Ageing Soc*. 2010;30(4):697.

31. Kim KB, Yun JH, Sok SR. Effects of individual reminiscence therapy on older adults' depression, morale and quality of life. *Taehan Kanho Hakhoe Chi* 2006;**36**(5):813–820.

32. Lok N, Bademli K, Selcuk-Tosun A. The effect of reminiscence therapy on cognitive functions, depression, and quality of life in Alzheimer patients: randomized controlled trial. *Int J Geriatr Psychiatry*. 2019;34:47–53.

33. Tadaka E, Kanagawa K. Effects of reminiscence group in elderly people with Alzheimer disease and vascular dementia in a community setting. *Geriatric Gerontology Int*. 2007;7(2):167–173.

34. Serrano Selva JP, Latorre Postigo JM, Ros Segura L, et al. Life review therapy using autobiographical retrieval practice for older adults with clinical depression. *Psicothema*. 2012;24(2):224–229.

35. Kuyken W, Brewin CR. Autobiographical memory functioning in depression and reports of early abuse. *J Abnorm Psychol*. 1995;**104**:585–591.

36. Elisa SM, Neville C, Scott T. The effectiveness of group reminiscence therapy for loneliness, anxiety and depression in older adults in long-term care: a systematic review. *Geriatr Nurs*. 2015;36:372–380.

37. Huang HC, Chen YT, Chen PY, et al. Reminiscence therapy improves cognitive functions and reduces depressive symptoms in elderly people with dementia: a meta-analysis of randomized controlled trials. *J Am Med Dir Assoc*. 2015;**16**(12):1087–1094.

38. Chiang KJ, Chu H, Chang HJ, et al. The effects of reminiscence therapy on psychological well-being, depression, and loneliness among the institutionalized aged. *Int J Geriatr Psychiatry*. 2010;25:380–388.

39, Karimi H, Dolatshahee B, Momeni K, et al. Effectiveness of integrative and instrumental reminiscence therapies on depression symptoms reduction in institutionalized older adults: an empirical study. *Aging Ment Health.* 2010;**14**:881–887.

40. Haslam C, Haslam SA, Jetten J, et al. The social treatment: the benefits of group interventions in residential care settings. *Psychol Aging.* 2010;**25**: 157–167.

41. Gibson F. *Reminiscence and life story work: a practice guide.* London: Jessica Kingsley Publishers; 2011.

42. Brody C, Samel V. Working with staff, families and residents in an institution: review of the literature. In: *Relevant issues and approaches for therapy. Strategies for therapy with the elderly. Living with hope and meaning.* New York: Springer; 2005. p. 41–56.

43. Cohen-Mansfield J, Marx M, Dakheel-Ali M, et al. Can agitated behavior of nursing home residents with dementia be prevented with the use of standardized stimuli? *J Am Geriatr Soc.* (2010);**58**(8):1459–1464.

44. Vink AC, Zuidersma M, Boersma F, et al. The effect of music therapy compared with general recreational activities in reducing agitation in people with dementia: a randomized controlled trial. *Int Geriatr Psychiatry.* (2013);**28**(10):1031–1038.

45. Cohen-Mansfield J, Dakheel-Ali M, Marx MS. Engagement in persons with dementia: the concept and its measurement. *Am J Geriatr Psychiatry.* 2009;**17**(4):299–307.

46. Cohen-Mansfield J, Marx MS, Thein K, et al. The impact of stimuli on affect in persons with dementia. *J Clin Psychiatry.* 2011;**72**(4):480–490.

47. Ballard C, Brown R, Fossey J, et al. Brief psychosocial therapy for the treatment of agitation in Alzheimer disease (the CALM-AD trial). *Am J Geriatr Psychiatry.* 2009;**17**(9):726–733.

48. Zhang HH, Liu PC, Ying J., et al. Evaluation of MESSAGE communication strategy combined with group reminiscence therapy on elders with mild cognitive impairment in long-term care facilities. *Int J Geriatr Psychiatry.* 2018;**33**(4):613–622.

49. Joosten-Weyn LW, Kessels RP, Olde Rikkert MG, et al. A cognitive behavioral group therapy for patients diagnosed with mild cognitive impairment and their significant others: feasibility and preliminary results. *Clin Rehabil.* 2008;**22**(8):731–740.

50. Cohen-Mansfield J, Hai T, Comishen M. Group engagement in persons with dementia: the concept and its measurement. *Psychiatry Research.* 2017;**251**:237–243.

51. Cohen-Mansfield J, Hirshfeld K, Gavendo R, et al. Activity-in-a-box for engaging persons with dementia in groups: implications for therapeutic recreation practice. *Am J Recreat Ther.* 2016;**15**(3):8–18.

52. Roos V, Malan L. The role of context and the interpersonal experience of loneliness among older people in a residential care facility. *Glob Health Action.* 2012;**5**:1–10.

53. Cheng ST. Dementia caregiver burden: a research update and critical analysis. *Curr Psychiatry Rep.* 2017;**19**(9):64.

54. Schulz R, Sherwood PR. Physical and mental health effects of family caregiving. *Am J Nurs.* 2008;**108**(9):23–27.

55. Greene VL, Monahan DJ. The effect of professionally guided care-giver support and education groups on institutionalized care receivers. *The Gerontologist.* 1987;**27**:716–72I.

56 Greene VL, Monahan DJ.The effect of a support and education program on stress and burden among family caregivers to frail elderly persons. *The Gerontologist.* 1989;**29**:472–480.

57. Haley WE.Group intervention for dementia family caregivers: a longitudinal perspective. *The Gerontologist.* 1989;**29**:481–483.

End-of-Life Issues

13

James Gerhart and Sandra Swantek

Introduction: Overview of the Last Stage of Life

As with all other stages of life, the last – the process and experience of death – occurs within a complex biopsychosocial context. Interacting systems, ranging from the cellular and physiologic to familial, cultural, and economic, shape related phenomenological experiences of personal meaning, fear, fatigue, and hope for transcendence. Acknowledging the many ways and times to die, medical advancements have greatly expanded life expectancies, and a substantial portion of the population lives with chronic illnesses that were previously acutely fatal. This chapter focuses specifically on the provision of psychotherapy for older adults experiencing dying processes that are protracted enough for them to contemplate their mortality, probable causes, aftermath, and other broader existential themes of their lives. This chapter examines the dying experience within the broad framework of evolutionary psychology, which aims to describe and explain the human condition, individual differences, and the individual life narrative based on principles of evolutionary theory.[1]

The biomedical sciences primarily sought and succeeded somewhat in delaying death. Death itself has been challenging to define, and a source of legal and ethical controversy.[2–4] Likewise, it has been difficult to demarcate the various processes and stages of dying and characterize the considerable individual differences in the psychological response to dying.[4] That said, some consensus exists that one enters into the dying process when the failure of one or more organ systems becomes irreversible. The subsequent failure of other systems, and the eventual failure of the cardio-respiratory system and the nervous system underpinning consciousness, leads to widespread cell death. Significant variation exists at the biological level, depending on the cause of death and the order in which systems fail. Further variation exists in the level and quality of consciousness and cognition, the manner in which individuals interpret their impending deaths, and the quality and meaning of their lives.

Psychiatrist Elisabeth Kübler-Ross observed that death is the ultimate psychological and existential mystery.[5] All organisms die, but the human species is unique in its ability to verbally construct the meaning of death, devise plans to forestall it, and in some cases hasten its arrival.[6] Despite a sometimes poignant awareness of eventual mortality, individuals often avoid and suppress awareness of the internal and external reminders of it, and so the breaking of bad news by a healthcare professional can be met with shock, acute stress, and even posttraumatic reactions by some patients. Rigid *experiential avoidance*, defined as the tendency to avoid, suppress, and minimize uncomfortable thoughts, emotions, and the situations that trigger them, has been implicated as a transdiagnostic vulnerability to psychopathology and psychological distress.[7] The extent to which patients access social supports, psychosocial care, and adequate pain and symptom management facilitates psychological adjustment. New evidence suggests that in the case of advanced cancer, efforts to palliate symptoms may not only enhance physical and psychological wellbeing but also extend survival.[8] Thus, it is crucial that patients have the opportunity to voice their worries, fears, and regrets, and palliate symptoms in ways consistent with their values

Setting the Stage

The purpose of this chapter is to assist clinicians in addressing the psychosocial concerns of patients approaching the end of life. The crucial question is what patients need to experience in order to have a sense of wellbeing during this final stage of living. In his classic developmental theory, Erikson and his colleagues postulated that older adults are impelled to reflect on life and find meaning, coherence, and wholeness regarding the course their lives have taken.[9] If this reflection unearths substantial regret or a lack of fulfillment and meaning, the older adult may experience despair, depression, and other adverse reactions. Specific sources of value, purpose, and meaning tend to be conceptual or symbolic, and are, some argue, freely chosen by the individual.[10] That said, an evolutionary framework of psychology argues that individuals are often motivated to navigate the social world through affiliation and attachments while also competing for status and achievements. At the end of life, patients may reflect on themes and patterns that connect them to others, and also find meaning and pride in the achievements and successes that set them apart from their peers.[1] This construction of meaning within an interpersonal framework also speaks to the eusocial nature of the human species. The management of stress and preservation of resources occur within social systems of increasing complexity regarding the dyad, the family, the community, and the culture.[11] Therefore, treatment approaches at the end of life may be considered within individual or larger social units.

Supporting the Individual: Reducing Discomforts and Sustaining Rewards

Stress arises in response to the actual or threatened loss of one's valued resources.[11] The physiological stress-response is likely an adaptation that functions to ward off acute threats, such as bodily harm, from adversaries and accidents via freeze-flight-and-fight responses. While patients may experience acute anxiety and anger, the process of dying in today's world tends to be much more protracted. Profound losses are salient in the case of chronic illness that limits activities. Attention is often disproportionately directed to the illness and related sources of stress including financial strain and social stigma.[12] Although stress responses may be normative and expected near the end of life, they are not necessarily adaptive and may perpetuate cycles of loss.

Patients facing the end of life may vary in their ability to remain engaged in the adaptive and meaningful activities of living. The behavioral model underpinning behavioral activation (BA) therapy argues that the loss of reinforcers or the stimuli that follow and maintain adaptive behaviors results in depressive behaviors such as cognitive rumination, withdrawal, and psychomotor retardation.[13,14] This model defines depression as the loss of engagement in the meaningful activities that bring pleasure. Therefore, it is crucial that patients have opportunities to increase and sustain social supports, hobbies, and other activities that produce rewards. Efforts must be made to mitigate adverse events, including pain, nausea, and social conflict, that punish or decrease engagement in adaptive behavior.

Behavioral activation fosters problem-solving, flexibility, and creative thinking, and encourages patients to identify their activity prescription through rewarding activities such as music, games, meals, spiritual practices, and visits or phone calls with loved ones that may be feasible despite pain, physical limitations, and other symptoms.[15]

Although palliative interventions and psychosocial care may benefit individual patients, those experiencing higher levels of depression and anxiety may be more reticent to seek services.[16] This paradox is consistent with studies showing that only a minority of individuals who stand to benefit engage in psychotherapy whether it be related to mental or life-threatening illness.[17] Even in cases where patients are reluctant to engage in individual treatment, bolstering external supports within the patient's social support system may be possible.

Supporting the Family: Promoting Self-Care

Real and threatened losses related to impending mortality are also salient for the family as the patient approaches the end of life. In addition to the threat of impending death of the patient, caregivers, spouses, and family often face substantial changes in their daily routines. Caregiving duties may be burdensome for those with their own health problems, particularly spouses of advanced age. Caregiving duties may also interfere with the parenting and work responsibilities of younger family members. Children within the family may be fearful and potentially frustrated with shifts in routines and the family dynamic.

Support of the dying patient includes encouraging family members to engage in self-care consistent with a BA model. Reminders, encouragement, and other prompts may be necessary to ensure that family members care for their health needs, including getting enough sleep, nutrition, and exercise. In family systems affected by trauma, family secrets, and financial tensions, the impending death of a loved one may bring conflicts to the surface or increase the intensity of an ongoing conflict. In this case, family therapy with an emphasis on social problem-solving therapy (PST)[18] may help family members identify salient problems, set reasonable goals, and approach current problems pragmatically and creatively. Other trauma-focused cognitive behavioral strategies may be useful for helping families navigate the end of life in the context of personal or shared trauma. Children struggling with change or anticipated loss may benefit from consultation with a Child Life Specialist.[19]

Activating the Community and Culture

Community supports should be activated when family support systems are threatened or strained. Access to palliative care and supportive services varies within the United States. These differences often relate to regional differences in personality, politics, and culture.[20] To the extent that formalized palliative care services are absent or insufficient, patients and their families may benefit from case management that connects them to senior centers, clubhouses, hospices, and other agencies that may provide resources and respite for caregivers, allowing them to attend to self-care and other duties. National organizations such as the American Cancer Society may assist in addressing practical needs such as transportation and copay relief. Mosques, parishes, churches, temples, and other religious groups in the community provide spiritual and religious support along with emotional and instrumental support. As with the family, flexible and creative problem-solving strategies may be of benefit for activating supports within the community.[18]

Cultural humility and self-reflection on the part of the clinician is warranted, as social scripts may impact how patients and families seek social support within their communities and culture. The patient's personal experiences and preferences should play a paramount role. For example, patients experiencing religious struggle who may benefit from spiritual care may be reticent to speak with religious leaders and chaplains. Other patients may be embarrassed to seek support from neighbors. As Kübler-Ross argued many years ago, clinicians should accept and respect patient preferences while recognizing that such preferences will sometimes conflict with the priorities, values, or clinical judgment of the clinician.[5] Clinicians must be discerning about whether to encourage patients and families to push through their feelings of embarrassment in order to seek support.

Sustaining and Restoring Meaning and Dignity in the Last Stage of Life

Humans and nonhumans share essential drives for food, shelter, and safety. Victor Frankl, a psychiatrist and existential thinker, argued that what makes humans different from other species is an additional drive to establish a sense of meaning.[21] Frankl's thinking grew out of his experience as a survivor of the Holocaust perpetrated by the Nazis. He noted that while culture shapes human meaning and value, it is social connectedness, work, spirituality, and love that bring meaning at the end of life.[21] Both classic and contemporary theories of psychology identify a shared central motive to affiliate with others while striving for status and resources.[1] The individual's life narrative and self-concept constructed around relationships, role, achievements, and other vital experiences bring meaning, even at the end of life. However, as people near death, they may encounter a myriad of problems that undermine their sense of dignity and personhood. Losses and suffering resulting from chronic illness and protracted dying may pose a significant threat to these sources of meaning. Profound suffering, in the form of pain, fatigue, or nausea, limits a person's ability to engage in social and occupational activities that once provided meaning and purpose. The individual's loss of control of the body and bodily functions has the potential to undermine the individual's sense of control, autonomy, and dignity. However, Frankl[21] asserted that suffering itself is a condition that allows for the discovery of meaning. To the extent that an individual can acknowledge and accept that life often entails unavoidable pain and distress, they are in a better position to avoid isolation and self-criticism, and to maintain engagement in meaningful activities and relationships.[10]

The awareness of impending death moves persons to seek transcendence and legacy. They may pursue transcendence by connecting to the values, beliefs, and practices of family, culture, and social grouping. Thus, while consciousness may cease at the end of life, central components of the self, including morals, values, dreams, and preferences, persist when they are shared socially with others.[22] The sharing of meaningful experiences and practices may be of psychological benefit to the patient, and may also impart information and motivation to guide the activity of future generations. Meaning-centered therapy[23] and dignity therapy[24] are two forms of therapy developed to assist patients in addressing the fundamental needs for meaning and relationship while managing anxieties and other negative emotions faced at the end of life. We describe these approaches below.

Meaning-Centered Therapy

Meaning-centered therapy is an educational intervention that explores patients' fundamental needs at the end of life while supporting them in identifying that which brings meaning to them. Developed by William Breitbart and directly influenced by the work of Victor Frankl, meaning-centered therapy is appropriate for both individual and group settings.

Individual treatment consists of seven 60-minute sessions, while the group format consists of eight 90-minute sessions – an abbreviated format serving the needs of patients receiving palliative care in the hospital is also available. Meaning-centered group psychotherapy (MCGP) is described as an educational intervention for patients that can be delivered over the course of eight sessions.[25,26] In each session, patients are encouraged to integrate the didactic content with personal experiences through a series of experiential exercises subsequently shared with fellow members. For instance, early sessions introduce information on meaning and the implications of cancer on meaning; patients are encouraged to reflect and write on topics that include instances in life where meaning was salient to them and to explore how cancer affected their sense of identity. As the group progresses, patients explore other aspects of meaning, including their accomplishments and the legacy they will leave for others. The sessions address the creative aspects of meaning derived through commitments and responsibilities to others. The sessions also support and seek to imbue patients with a sense of courage in their reflections on such challenges and threats to meaning as activity limitations, mortality, and unfinished business. In randomized trials, MCGP produced outcomes superior to alternative treatments, such as supportive group therapy.[27] Moreover, mediation analysis suggests that increases in meaning and peace explain the impact of MCGP on depression and other treatment outcomes.[27]

Dignity Therapy

Chochinov and colleagues developed dignity therapy to guide patients' reflections on meaningful events in their lives with the goal of increasing dignity and purpose for patients with terminal illnesses and life expectancies of six months or less.[24] Dignity therapy also draws from the work of Victor Frankl. In reflecting on the death of his wife during the Holocaust, Frankl recognized and found some comfort in the certitude of past events. Acknowledging that memory is fallible, Frankl found that reflection on prior joyous and satisfying events could bring a sense of meaning and purpose to bear in the present and future.[21]

Dignity therapy supports patients as they actively reflect on the purpose inherent in their lives.[24] This reflection produces a narrative. In turn, this life narrative or legacy document is shared with loved ones. Patients are guided to reflect on central themes of purpose and meaning.[28] The questions prompt patients to consider their social, familial, and occupational roles, and to offer wisdom and encouragement to family members.

As with other classic and contemporary approaches to psychotherapy, dignity therapy emphasizes the quality of the therapeutic interaction or the working alliance.[24] Clinicians are encouraged to be attentive, curious and empathic as patients develop their legacy document. Meaning is developed and enhanced through reflection on memories, future dreams for families, and also through the care, support, and validation provided by the clinician's acceptance of the patient in the present moment.

Explicit flexibility makes dignity therapy distinct from some other psychotherapies. The clinician implementing dignity therapy may be a physician, nurse, or other healthcare professional. The bedside is commonly the setting for this treatment. Recognizing the uncertainty inherent to the end of life, the timeline for dignity therapy is brief and open-ended. The intervention can be delivered during a single session or developed incrementally over several sessions.

Evidence for the efficacy of dignity therapy is growing, but the results are mixed. In a review of 28 studies, Martinez and colleagues found 5 randomized control trials (RCTs) testing dignity therapy.[29] Patients experiencing higher levels of distress appeared to be more responsive to treatment; two RCTs that included patients with high levels of baseline distress showed improvements in anxiety. One of these two trials also showed a decrease in depression. The studies found dignity therapy to be associated with improved measures of quality of life, reduced sadness, and enhanced spiritual wellbeing. Patients and families perceived the intervention as helpful.

Other Psychotherapeutic Approaches Employed in Hospice

Whereas the bulk of the research on evidence-based interventions at the end of life has centered on dignity therapy and meaning-centered therapy, other approaches are also implemented in the context of Hospice and end-of-life care. Many of the theoretical models fall under the umbrella of cognitive behavioral therapy (CBT), which aims to ease distress through awareness and modification of unhelpful or maladaptive thought processes and other behaviors. Anderson, Watson, and Davidson implemented CBT across 3–4 sessions with 11 patients in Hospice.[30] Patients utilized thought diaries, challenged unhelpful cognitions, practiced relaxation, and set goals. This small trial demonstrated significant reductions in depression and anxiety, and high patient satisfaction with the program. Similar small-scale studies investigated the feasibility of implementing mindfulness-based interventions for patients with terminal cancer.[31] In another study, patients and family members randomized to a 5-minute mindfulness intervention reported reductions in distress when compared to a control condition where patients were listened to by others.[32] Other approaches to reducing distress in terminally ill individuals have included music therapy[33] and spiritual care.[34]

Mechanisms of Change

The growth of evidence-based psychotherapies led to increased recognition that interventions developed around distinct theoretical models may produce similar outcomes when tested with group designs.[35,36] Some findings suggest that this also may be the case with end-of-life care. If treatments based on different theories of human behavior operate similarly, the question remains: Why do different interventions produce similar outcomes? Common factors cited in the literature include the importance of the therapeutic alliance, client expectation, and clinician skill in fostering change.[36] However, the possibility remains that different approaches could work equally well for different reasons and that the precise mechanisms that facilitate therapeutic change are still not well understood.[37–39] As noted previously, some evidence suggests that improvements in depression resulting from MCGP may be explained by an increased sense of meaning and peace.[27] This analysis points to increased meaning as an essential mechanism to target as part of intervention at the end of life.

When Treatments Harm

To the extent that terminal illness may be traumatic, there is concern that unwarranted intervention could increase symptoms of traumatic stress and depression. Similar to early work on critical incident stress debriefing, which demonstrated the potential for increasing trauma-related distress in some samples, some research has found that routine palliative care consultation could lead to increased post-traumatic stress disorder (PTSD) symptoms among family members.[40] Statistically nonsignificant increases in anxiety observed in dignity therapy are nevertheless distressing for the individual experiencing the anxiety. Thus, good practice requires evaluating, as much as is feasible, the appropriateness of psychotherapy for patients, careful monitoring of the therapy processes, patient satisfaction, and outcome.

Clinician Wellbeing and End-of-Life Care

Research into the common factors of psychotherapy highlights several contextual factors that facilitate treatment outcomes, including clinician empathy and the alliance between the clinician and the patient. At the end of life, taking the perspective of patients often means that clinicians become more aware of their own mortality and the impermanence of relationships in both their personal and professional experience. Although considerably more research is needed to understand the impact on mental health clinicians working in end-of-life care, current assumptions are that clinician wellbeing in relation to care for individuals with serious and life-threatening illnesses depends in part on personal factors such as personality traits and emotion regulation strategies.[41,42] Clinicians working in these settings also stand to benefit from professional and organizational supports, such as supervision, networking, and occupational social supports.[43] Although some interventions have been developed to support the coping of healthcare professionals in palliative care and hospice settings, more research is needed.[44] Mindfulness and acceptance-based interventions may be promising for reducing symptoms of depression and burnout in some clinicians.[45,46]

Conclusions

As medical science extends the period of time that persons with chronic medical illness survive, increasing numbers of adults will live with the knowledge that they have illnesses that may be treated but not cured. While some persons may choose to ignore their mortality, for others the awareness of the closeness of death will create a need to come to terms with life issues previously left unresolved. Cognitive therapy-based interventions show benefit for persons with terminal illness and their families. Clinicians familiar with these interventions have additional tools to support patients in realizing comfort and resolution at the end of life. As with any intervention, the clinician must adapt treatment to the particular biopsychosocial needs of the patient and family. Not all patients or families will want to take part in end-of-life therapy. Studies suggesting increased anxiety or PTSD for some participants highlight how little is known about the precise mechanisms that facilitate therapeutic change and the need for additional investigation. The clinician is encouraged to make a careful clinical assessment prior to initiating end-of-life therapy and adjust treatment to the patient.

References

1. McAdams DP, Pals JL. A new big five: fundamental principles for an integrative science of personality. *Am Psychol.* 2006;61(3):204–217.

2. President's Commission for the Study of Ethical Problems in Medicine and Biomedical and Behavioral Research. US Code Annot US. 1982;Title42 Sect. 300v as added 1978. PMID: 12041401

3. Burkle CM, Sharp RR, Wijdicks EF. Why brain death is considered death and why there should be no confusion. *Neurology.* 2014;83(16):1464–1469.

4. Hui D, Nooruddin Z, Didwaniya N, et al. Concepts and definitions for "actively dying," "end of life," "terminally ill," "terminal care," and "transition of care": a systematic review. *J Pain Symptom Manage.* 2014;47(1):77–89. PMID: 23796586

5. Kübler-Ross E, Wessler S, Avioli L V. On death and dying. *JAMA.* 1972;221 (2):174–179.

6. Törneke, NL, Carmen Salas SV. Rule-governed behavior and psychological problems. *Int J Psychol Psychol Ther.* 2008;8 (2):141–156.

7. Monestès J-L, Karekla M, Jacobs N, et al. Experiential avoidance as a common psychological process in European cultures. *Eur J Psychol Assess.* 2018;34(4):247–257. doi/10.1027/1015-5759/a000327

8. Hoerger M, Wayser GR, Schwing G, Suzuki A, Perry LM. Impact of interdisciplinary outpatient specialty palliative care on survival and quality of life in adults with advanced cancer: a meta-analysis of randomized controlled trials. *Ann Behav Med.* 2018 Sept 28. Retrieved from: www.academic.oup.com/abm/advance-article/doi/10.1093/abm/kay077/5108509 (March 3, 2019).

9. Erikson EH, Erickson JM, Kivnick HQ. *Vital involvement in old age.* New York: WW Norton; 1989.

10. Hayes SC, Strosahl K, Wilson KG. *Acceptance and commitment therapy : the process and practice of mindful change.* 2nd ed. New York: Guilford Press; 2012.

11. Hobfoll SE. *Stress, culture, and community: the psychology and philosophy of stress.* Boston: Springer; 1998.

12. Hobfoll SE, Tirone V, Holmgreen L, Gerhart J. *Conservation of resources theory applied to major stress. Stress: concepts, cognition, emotion, and behavior .* In: Fink G, editor. *Vol 1. Stress: concepts, cognition, emotion and behavior.* San Diego, CA: Elsevier; 2016. p. 65–71.

13. Ferster CB. A functional analysis of depression. *Am Psychol.* 1973;28 (10):857–870.

14. Martell CR, Addis M, Dimidjian S. Finding the action in behavioral activation: the search for empirically supported interventions and mechanisms of change. In: Hayes SC, Follette VM, Linehan MM, editors. *Mindfulness and acceptance: expanding the cognitive-behavioral tradition.* New York: Guilford Press; 2004. p. 152–167.

15. Swantek S, Fairchild M, Smith M, Gollan J. Innovative treatment of geriatric depression: a feasibility study. *Am J Geriatr Psychiatry.* 2013;21(3):S132.

16. Gerhart J, Asvat Y, Lattie E, et al. Distress, delay of gratification and preference for palliative care in men with prostate cancer. *Psychooncology.* 2016;25(1):91–96.

17. Van Scheppingen C, Schroevers MJ, Pool G, et al. Is implementing screening for distress an efficient means to recruit patients to a psychological intervention trial? *Psychooncology.* 2014;23(5):516–523.

18. Nezu AM, Nezu CM, Felgoise SH, et al. Project Genesis: assessing the efficacy of problem-solving therapy for distressed adult cancer patients. *J Consult Clin Psychol.* 2003;71(6):1036–1048.

19. Committee on Hospital Care and Child Life Council. Child life services. *Pediatrics.* 2014;133(5):e1471–e1478.

20. Hoerger M, Perry LM, Korotkin BD, et al. Statewide differences in personality associated with geographic disparities in access to palliative care: findings on openness. *J Palliat Med [Preprint].* 2019. doi:10.1089/jpm.2-18.0206

21. Frankl VE. *Man's Search for meaning: an introduction to logotherapy.* New York: Simon and Schuster; 1959.

22. Burke BL, Martens A, Faucher EH. Two decades of terror management theory: a meta-analysis of mortality salience research. *Personal Soc Psychol Rev.* 2010;14 (2):155–195.

23. Breitbart W, Poppito S, Rosenfeld B, et al. Pilot randomized controlled trial of individual meaning-centered

psychotherapy for patients with advanced cancer. *J Clin Oncol.* 2012;30 (12):1304–1309.

24. Chochinov HM, Hack T, Hassard T, et al. Dignity therapy: a novel psychotherapeutic intervention for patients near the end of life. *J Clin Oncol.* 2005;23(24):5520–5525.

25. Breitbart WS, Poppito SR. *Individual meaning-centered psychotherapy for patients with advanced cancer: a treatment manual.* New York: Oxford University Press; 2014.

26. Breitbart W, Applebaum A. Meaning-centered group psychotherapy. In: Watson M, Kisante DW, editors. *Handbook of psychotherapy in cancer care.* Hoboken, NJ: John Wiley & Sons; 2011. p. 137–148.

27. Rosenfeld B, Cham H, Pessin H, Breitbart W. Why is meaning-centered group psychotherapy (MCGP) effective? Enhanced sense of meaning as the mechanism of change for advanced cancer patients. *Psychooncology.* 2018;27 (2):654–660.

28. Chochinov HM, Kristjanson LJ, Breitbart W, et al. Effect of dignity therapy on distress and end-of-life experience in terminally ill patients: a randomised controlled trial. *Lancet Oncol.* 2011;12 (8):753–762.

29. Martínez M, Arantzamendi M, Belar A, et al. "Dignity therapy," a promising intervention in palliative care: a comprehensive systematic literature review. *Palliat Med.* 2017 Jun 26;31 (6):492–509.

30. Anderson T, Watson M, Davidson R. The use of cognitive behavioural therapy techniques for anxiety and depression in hospice patients: a feasibility study. *Palliat Med.* 2008;22(7):814–821.

31. Chadwick P, Newell T, Skinner C. Mindfulness groups in palliative care: a pilot qualitative study. *Spiritual Heal Int.* 2008;9(3):135–144.

32. Ng CG, Lai KT, Tan SB, Sulaiman AH, Zainal NZ. The effect of 5 minutes of mindful breathing to the perception of distress and physiological responses in palliative care cancer patients: a randomized controlled study. *J Palliat Med.* 2016;19(9):917–924.

33. Cadwalader A, Orellano S, Tanguay C, Roshan R. The effects of a single session of music therapy on the agitated behaviors of patients receiving hospice care. *J Palliat Med.* 2016;19(8):870–873.

34. Epstein-Peterson ZD, Sullivan AJ, Enzinger AC, et al. Examining forms of spiritual care provided in the advanced cancer setting. *Am J Hosp Palliat Med.* 2015;32 (7):750–757.

35. Messer SB, Wampold BE. Let's face facts: common factors are more potent than specific therapy ingredients. *Clinical Psychology: Science and Practice.* 2002;9 (1):21.

36. Wampold BE. How important are the common factors in psychotherapy? *An update. World Psychiatry.* 2015;14 (3):270–271.

37. Kazdin AE. Understanding how and why psychotherapy leads to change. *Psychother Res.* 2009;19(4–5):418–428.

38. Kazdin AE. Moderators, mediators and mechanisms of change in psychotherapy. In: Lutz W, Knox S, editors. *Quantitative and qualitative methods in psychotherapy research.* New York: Routledge/Taylor & Francis; 2014. p. 87–101.

39. Kazdin AE. Treatment outcomes, common factors, and continued neglect of mechanisms of change. *Clin Psychol Sci Pract.* 2005;12(2):184–188.

40. Carson SS, Cox CE, Wallenstein S, et al. Effect of palliative care-led meetings for families of patients with chronic critical illness. *JAMA.* 2016;316(1): 51–52.

41. Gerhart J, Vaclavik E, Lillis TA, et al. A daily diary study of posttraumatic stress, experiential avoidance, and emotional lability among inpatient nurses. *Psychooncology.* 2018;27(3):1068–1071.

42. O'Mahony S, Gerhart JI, Grosse J, Abrams I, Levy MM. Posttraumatic stress symptoms in palliative care professionals seeking mindfulness training: prevalence and vulnerability. *Palliat Med.* 2016;30 (2):189–192.

43. Najjar N, Davis LW, Beck-Coon K, Carney DC. Compassion fatigue. *J Health Psychol.* 2009;14(2):267–277.

44. Hill RC, Dempster M, Donnelly M, McCorry NK. Improving the wellbeing of staff who work in palliative care settings: a systematic review of psychosocial interventions. *Palliative Medicine.* 2016;30 (9):825–833.

45. O'Mahony S, Gerhart J, Abrams I, et al. A multimodal mindfulness training to address mental health symptoms in providers who care for and interact with children in relation to end-of-life care. *Am J Hosp Palliat Med.* 2017;34 (9):838–843.

46. Gerhart J, O'Mahony S, Abrams I, et al. A pilot test of a mindfulness-based communication training to enhance resilience in palliative care professionals. *J Context Behav Sci.* 2016;5 (2):89–96.

Index